AMERICAN JOURNAL of PUBLIC HEALTH
JUNE 2024
Issue 6

AJPH

A PUBLICATION OF THE
AMERICAN PUBLIC HEALTH ASSOCIATION

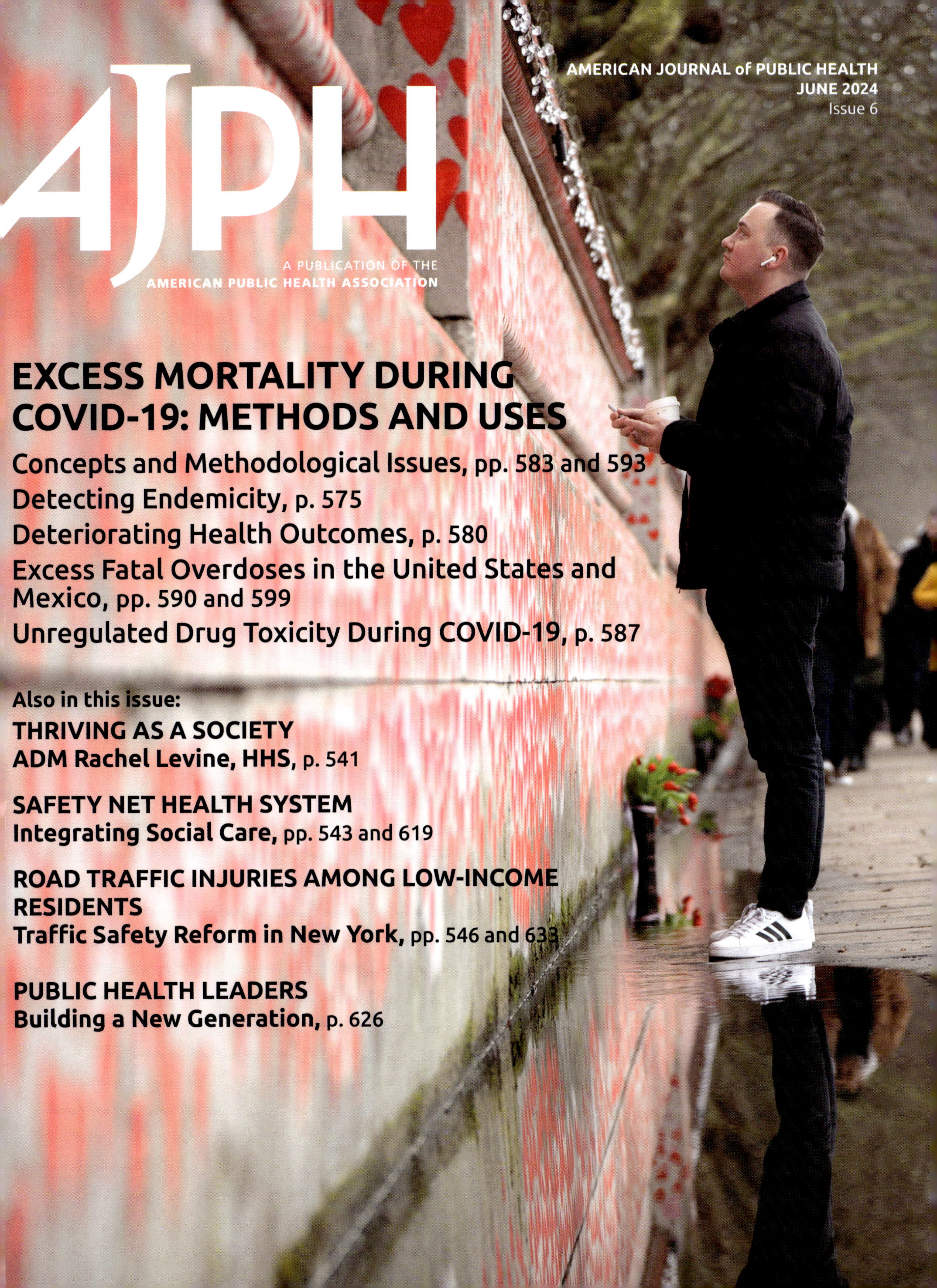

EXCESS MORTALITY DURING COVID-19: METHODS AND USES

Concepts and Methodological Issues, pp. 583 and 593
Detecting Endemicity, p. 575
Deteriorating Health Outcomes, p. 580
Excess Fatal Overdoses in the United States and Mexico, pp. 590 and 599
Unregulated Drug Toxicity During COVID-19, p. 587

Also in this issue:

THRIVING AS A SOCIETY
ADM Rachel Levine, HHS, p. 541

SAFETY NET HEALTH SYSTEM
Integrating Social Care, pp. 543 and 619

ROAD TRAFFIC INJURIES AMONG LOW-INCOME RESIDENTS
Traffic Safety Reform in New York, pp. 546 and 633

PUBLIC HEALTH LEADERS
Building a New Generation, p. 626

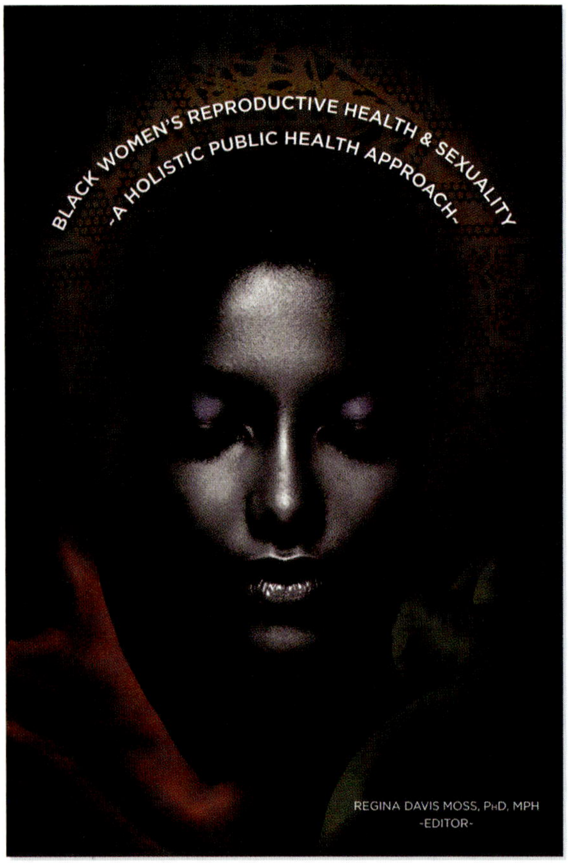

Black Women's Reproductive Health and Sexuality: A Holistic Public Health Approach

Edited by Regina Moss Davis, PhD, MPH

978-0-87553-340-7, 2023, 450 PP, SOFTCOVER

Reproductive health and sexual well-being are important parts of human health. But for Black women, research and education tend to focus on negative risks and outcomes. *Black Women's Reproductive Health and Sexuality: A Holistic Public Health Approach* offers a comprehensive look at the determinants of Black women's reproductive health and sexuality and shares evidence-based programs, policies, and promising solutions that support Black women in leading healthy and safe lives.

APHABOOKSTORE.ORG

APHA PRESS

AN IMPRINT OF AMERICAN PUBLIC HEALTH ASSOCIATION

APHA
AMERICAN PUBLIC HEALTH ASSOCIATION
For science. For action. For health.

AJPH®, published monthly, is the official Journal of the American Public Health Association®, 800 I St NW, Washington, DC 20001-3710; (202) 777- APHA; TDD (202) 777-2500. APHA is a nongovernmental professional society founded in 1872, representing all disciplines and specialties in public health.

The *American Journal of Public Health*® (*AJPH*) (print ISSN: 0090-0036; electronic ISSN: 1541- 0048), first published in 1911, is the official journal of the American Public Health Association® (APHA). The oldest and largest organization of public health professionals in the world, APHA represents approximately 30 000 members from more than 50 occupations of public health.

Submissions: Visit www.editorialmanager.com/ajph or ajph.edmgr.com for online manuscript preparation and submission guidelines. Contributions of original unpublished research, social science analyses, scholarly essays, critical commentaries, departments, and letters to the editor are welcome. Questions? Write ajph.submissions@apha.org or call APHA at (202) 777-2469.

Print plus online subscriptions: Institutional price (print copy with online access for a single institution and all authorized users, regardless of geographic location) varies by size of organization and ranges from $993–$1445 for US organizations, and $1073–$1526 for international organizations (air delivery); multiple campuses not permitted without special arrangement. Details of the tiered pricing system at https://subscriptionoffice.com/pages/apha-landing-page. To order, write apha.subscriptions@apha.org.

Online-only subscriptions: Institutional price for one institution and its authorized users (regardless of geographic location) is $878–$1307. To order, write apha.subscriptions@apha.org. For academic consortia or multisite corporate subscriptions, contact apha.subscriptions@apha.org.

Print-only subscriptions: Institutional price is US $701, $782 international.

Back print issues: A limited number of print issues are for sale. Single copies are US $49, $55 international (air delivery). Shipping included; prepay only. To order, write apha.subscriptions@apha.org.

Reprints: For prices and ordering information on 50 or more reprints, check the Reprints section at www.ajph.org. To order smaller quantities of reprints (rush delivery), use the "Purchase Article" link on the article site itself.

Electronic access: Online articles more than 10 years old are available free for personal use at www.ajph.org. Recent articles are available through pay-per-view: single PDF article for $24, single issue access for 24 hours for $33, or entire site access for 24 hours for $38.

Postal information: Periodicals postage paid at Washington, DC, and additional mailing offices. Postmaster: Send address changes to American Journal of Public Health, 800 I St NW, Washington, DC 20001-3710.

Address changes: Send to AJPH, Membership Department (members) or AJPH Subscriptions (subscribers), APHA, 800 I St NW, Washington, DC 20001-3710. Or write to membership.mail@apha. org (members) or apha.subscriptions@apha.org (subscribers).

Indexes: Publications that index or abstract articles from AJPH include the following: Ageline, Assia (Applied Social Science Index and Abstracts), Biological Abstracts, Chemical Abstracts, CINAHL, Criminal Justice Abstracts, EMBASE, EMCare, Environmental Abstracts, e-psyche, ERIC, ETOH (Alcohol and Alcohol Problems Science Database), Excerpta Medica, Food Science and Technology, General Science Index, Grateful Med, Hospital Literature Index, Human Resources Abstracts, International Pharmaceutical Abstracts (IPA), Medline, Physical Education Index, Pollution Abstracts, Psychological Abstracts, PsychINFO, Safety Science Abstracts, Sage Family Studies Abstracts, Sage Human Resources Abstracts, Science Citation Index, SCOPUS, SIIC Data Bases, Social Work Research and Abstracts, and Statistical Reference Index (SRI)/LexisNexis.

Medscape Publishers' Circle

AJPH

A PUBLICATION OF THE
AMERICAN PUBLIC HEALTH ASSOCIATION

COVER: People write names on the *National Covid Memorial Wall* on the Thames Path in Westminster, London, UK, for speeches and a minute's silence on the National Day of Reflection, in honor of those who died of COVID-19. Every hand-painted heart on the *Wall* represents a life that was lost to COVID-19 in the United Kingdom. Picture date: Sunday, March 3, 2024.

Cover concept and selection by Aleisha Kropf. Photo by James Manning/PA Images via Getty Images. Printed with permission.

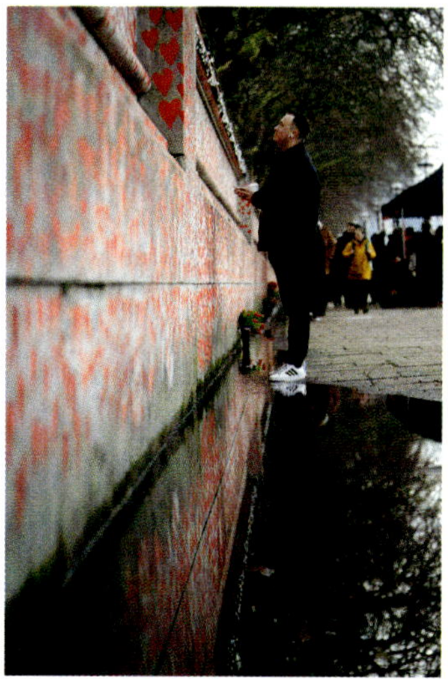

APHA
AMERICAN PUBLIC HEALTH ASSOCIATION
For science. For action. For health.

Promoting public health research, policy, practice, and education is the *AJPH* mission. As we widen our scope to embrace global issues, we also sharpen our focus to support the needs of public health practitioners. We invite contributions of original unpublished research, opinion and commentary, and letters to the editor.

The *Journal* is printed on acid-free recycled paper.

OPEN ACCESS   ONLINE ONLY   PODCAST   DATA SUPPLEMENT AVAILABLE

EDITOR'S CHOICE

541 Driving Change and Promoting Action to Thrive as a Society: Moving Social Determinants Into Unifying Action by Focusing on the Vital Conditions
R. L. Levine

OPINIONS, IDEAS, & PRACTICE

EDITORIALS

543 Integrating Social Care and Medical Care: From the Why to the How and Back Again
M. Silberberg

546 Building Momentum for a Safe System Approach to Reduce Road Traffic Injuries in the United States
J. P. Ehsani, G. Dolce, and J. P. Michael

548 Housing Ends Homelessness
J. D. Bamberger

550 Cannabis and Alcohol Involvement in Motor Vehicle Crashes: Reflections in the Era of Legalization
M. Asbridge and J. Brubacher

553 Disparities in Overdose Deaths: Looking Back at Larochelle and Colleagues' 2021 Paper
N. D. Volkow, B. Han, and R. K. Chandler

556 Life Expectancy in the United States: A Public Health of Consequence, June 2024
F. Kapadia

PERSPECTIVES

559 Public Health Legal Protections in an Era of Artificial Intelligence
J. G. Hodge Jr, J. L. Piatt, E. N. White, and L. O. Gostin

564 On the Appearance and Disappearance of Difficult Medical Histories: What Does It Take to Sustain Public Memory?
S. M. Reverby and A. Moran-Thomas

NOTES FROM THE FIELD

569 Barriers to and Facilitators of Pediatric Vaccination Reporting in Four US States, 2023
S. Israelsen-Hartley and N. A. Boucher

EXCESS MORTALITY CALCULATIONS: METHODS AND USES

575 On Detecting Endemicity: Insights from All-Cause Mortality Patterns During Epidemic Transitions
J. S. Faust

580 Malignant Neglect: Accounting for Public Disinterest in Deteriorating Health Outcomes in the United States
S. H. Woolf

583 Excess Mortality as a Tool to Monitor the Evolution of Health Emergencies: Choices, Challenges, and Future Directions
E. Paglino and A. C. Stokes

587 Local Impact From International Crises: Unregulated Drug Toxicity During the COVID-19 Pandemic in British Columbia, Canada
S. Tobias, J. A. Buxton, and L. Ti

590 Overdose and COVID-19 in Baja California, Mexico: The Need for New Methodologies for Understanding Local Trends
J. Arredondo Sanchez Lira and D. Goodman-Meza

RESEARCH & ANALYSIS

EXCESS MORTALITY CALCULATIONS: METHODS AND USES

593 Excess Mortality Calculations to Assess the Impact of the COVID-19 Pandemic: Concepts and Methodological Issues
J. P. Vandenbroucke and N. Pearce

599 Excess Fatal Overdoses in the United States During the COVID-19 Pandemic by Geography and Substance Type: March 2020–August 2021
J. Chandra, M-L. Charpignon, A. Bhaskar, A. Therriault, Y-H. Chen, A. Mooney, M. A. Dahleh, M. V. Kiang, and F. Dominici

HISTORY

610 First Decade of Supportive Services for Veteran Families Program and Homelessness, 2012–2022
R. Wilkinson, T. Byrne, R. G. Cowden K. N G. Long, J. H. Kuhn, H. K. Koh, and J. Tsai

POLICY

619 Building the Infrastructure to Integrate Social Care in a Safety Net Health System
C. M. Callahan, A. Carter, H. S. Carty D. O. Clark, T. Grain, S. L. Grant K. McElroy-Jones, D. Reinoso, and L. E. Harris

626 Building a New Generation of Public Health Leaders Forged in a Public Health Crisis
S. C. Helm-Murtagh and P. C. Erwin

SURVEILLANCE

633 Major Traffic Safety Reform and Road Traffic Injuries Among Low-Income New York Residents, 2009–2021
K. L. Dragan and S. A. Glied

OPEN-THEMED RESEARCH

642 Causes of Death in the Presence of Law Enforcement in Johnson County, Iowa, 2011–2020
A. M. L. Rempel, J. E. Persons, K. Bengtson, and M. B. Nashelsky

BACKMATTER

ERRATA

651 Erratum In: "Impact of a Permitless Concealed Firearm Carry Law in West Virginia, 1999–2015 and 2016–2020"

652 Erratum In: "Addressing Health Care Workers' Mental Health: A Systematic Review of Evidence-Based Interventions and Current Positives"

OTHER DEPARTMENTS

656 Subscription Form

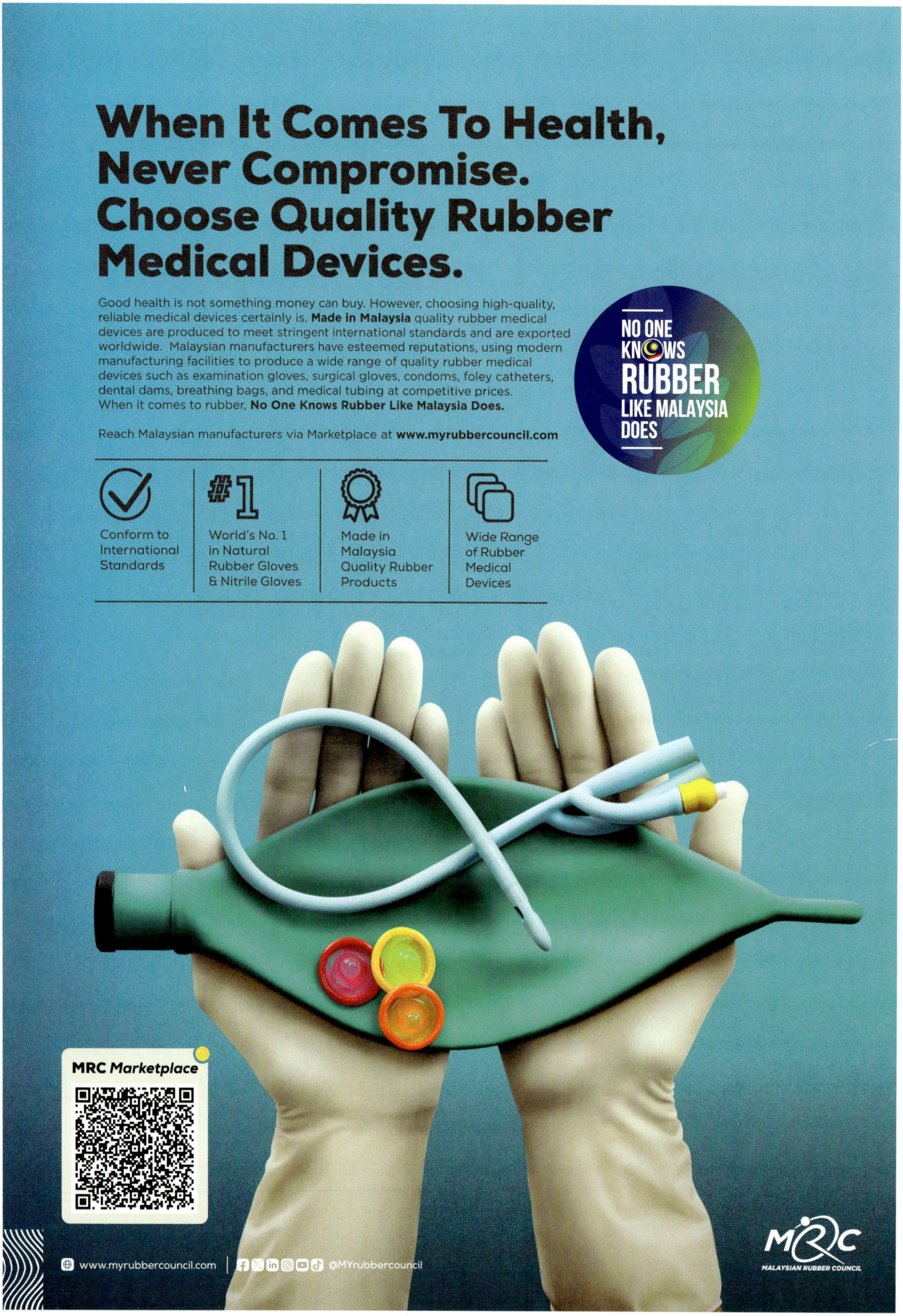
When It Comes To Health, Never Compromise. Choose Quality Rubber Medical Devices.
Good health is not something money can buy. However, choosing high-quality, reliable medical devices certainly is. **Made in Malaysia** quality rubber medical devices are produced to meet stringent international standards and are exported worldwide. Malaysian manufacturers have esteemed reputations, using modern manufacturing facilities to produce a wide range of quality rubber medical devices such as examination gloves, surgical gloves, condoms, foley catheters, dental dams, breathing bags, and medical tubing at competitive prices. When it comes to rubber, **No One Knows Rubber Like Malaysia Does.**
Reach Malaysian manufacturers via Marketplace at **www.myrubbercouncil.com**
NO ONE KNOWS RUBBER LIKE MALAYSIA DOES
Conform to International Standards
#1
World's No. 1 in Natural Rubber Gloves & Nitrile Gloves
Made in Malaysia Quality Rubber Products
Wide Range of Rubber Medical Devices
MRC Marketplace
www.myrubbercouncil.com
@MYrubbercouncil
MRC
MALAYSIAN RUBBER COUNCIL

Driving Change and Promoting Action to Thrive as a Society: Moving Social Determinants Into Unifying Action by Focusing on the Vital Conditions

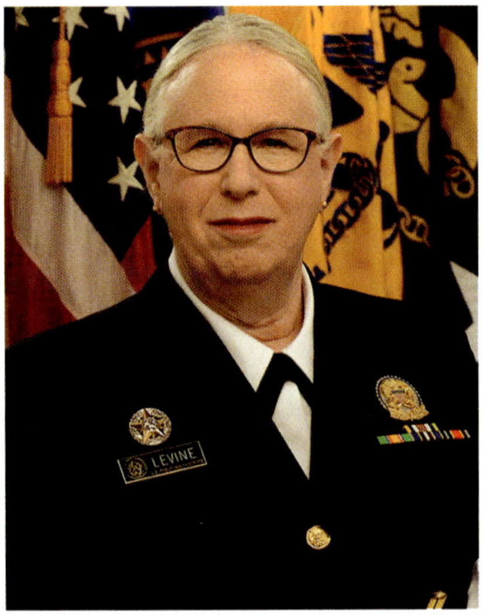

Rachel L. Levine, ADM, MD
Assistant Secretary for Health,
US Public Health Service
US Department of Health and Human Services

As public health practitioners, we have an opportunity to reposition our collective resources and expertise to support all people in every community as they seek to improve their well-being and ability to thrive. We must move beyond preventing disease to promoting thriving.

The US Department of Health and Human Services (HHS) is committed to integrating equity in programs and policies and creating the conditions for individuals and communities to thrive. As the assistant secretary for health, I champion two national initiatives that complement one another and call for action to resolve vulnerabilities and build capabilities that eliminate drivers of disparities, ultimately improving well-being. Healthy People 2030, the nation's 10-year foundational health plan, sets a vision for "a society in which all people can achieve their full potential for health and well-being across the lifespan" (https://bit.ly/3U1GBRo). People & Places Thriving (https://bit.ly/3VNHXk7) articulates actions that will transform historically disparate and reactive systems to harmonize resources so that we can strengthen resilience and achieve thriving.

We have the potential for catalytic action when we understand and use our

Continued on page 542...

HISTORY CORNER

47 YEARS AGO

Census Errors on Life Table Estimates and Black Mortality

Death statistics are generally considered accurate and complete, at least for most practical purposes, including life table construction, although it is important to note that a national death registration test has never been conducted. Inferences concerning the quality of death statistics are frequently drawn from the presumed diligence of medical examiners and funeral directors in following state public health codes which require the filing of a death certificate prior to the disposal of a body. These influences must be interpreted with some caution, however, because they tend to focus on the completeness of death registration rather than the accuracy of information reported on the death certificate. The basic demographic items on the certificate which are pertinent to life table construction are age, sex, and race. According to the National Center for Health Statistics, the only preliminary adjustment of the death statistics used to construct the most recent decennial life tables involves the prorated allocation of a relatively small number of deaths for which age at death was not stated on the certificate. Such an adjustment is standard procedure, but it does not address the accuracy with which age information is reported.

From *AJPH*, September 1977, p. 867

AJPH June 2024, Vol. 114, No. 6

resources as unified tools. Together, Healthy People and People & Places Thriving create the opportunity for employing ever-evolving insights into guiding how we braid our resources to foster powerful action that advances equitable resilience. Since its inception in 1979, Healthy People has set data-driven, national objectives. Many of these objectives address social determinants of health (SDOH): the conditions in which people are born, live, learn, work, play, worship, and age (https://bit.ly/4cFh9sm). Healthy People has tracked SDOH and has amassed evidence toward understanding, measuring, and acting on the drivers of health and well-being. Evidence demonstrates that addressing disparities requires shifting from a focus on individual, reactive, and prescriptive solutions to one on communal strengths and system capabilities that support individuals. Using those social determinants to common benefit requires that partners act beyond the health system.

People & Places Thriving is guided by the vital conditions for health, well-being, and justice framework (https://bit.ly/43L2fwH). The framework supports unifying action, as demonstrated in the initiative's recommendations (https://bit.ly/3VNHXk7). It evolved from the SDOH framework and articulates foundational capabilities of systems that form the building blocks for greater thriving in positive terms. To meet underlying needs, the vital conditions can be achieved only through collective resources and focus.

In examining the intersection of Healthy People, the SDOH framework, and the vital conditions framework, we see numerous linkages frequently used in policies and programs that offer potential opportunities to strengthen systems and capabilities that influence a range of social drivers. What's more, the frameworks can work in a complementary way to both identify the essential elements necessary to create thriving communities and address vulnerabilities.

For its part, HHS continues investing in work related to well-being research, language, and measurement, and we are championing partnerships across governmental and civil society sectors to align investments and build connections to foster needed change. This work grows more critical and complex by the day but is imperative for driving change, promoting action, and ultimately enhancing thriving. Working through the principle of shared stewardship, we collaborate, work from agreed on concepts and language, design multisolving solutions, and navigate this terrain with a common aspiration. Working in this way strengthens all our respective efforts—both as people and as professionals.

Complex problems are often easier to solve collectively than individually. We are all partners in promoting thriving, whether we know it in such terms or not. By working together to promote equity, we can ensure that all individuals and communities have the opportunity to thrive. I invite you to join me to align our focus, investments, and strategies that make multisystem solutions possible, both inside and outside of government. Together, we can thrive as a society. AJPH

DOI: https://doi.org/10.2105/AJPH.2024.307679

HISTORY CORNER

103 YEARS AGO

A Third Measuring Rod in Mortality Rates

Crude mortality rates, as shown by the Bureau of the Census, are in general measurable by the amounts of the filth-borne diseases, plus the respiratory diseases, plus a constant of 5.5, which latter figure was expressed as irreducible. . . . A study of the vital statistics over the years recorded shows that the constant 5.5 in the cities of the older registration area, and states as well, is year after year generally approximated by the sum of the amounts of the rates for cancer, violence, and of all other diseases. Using the rates for all other diseases multiplied by the constant 2.4, we have very generally for the various years and for all areas or specific parts of the registration area that measure of the previously used figure 5.5 which fulfills the following conditions. 1. Takes up the discrepancies of lower recorded over higher estimated rates. 2. Explains crude mortality rates of the country under 5 per 1,000 population. 3. Would seem to be an indicator of where a portion of one of the other measuring rods (of filth-borne diseases, for example) is erroneously contained.

From *AJPH*, October 1921, pp. 917–919

Integrating Social Care and Medical Care: From the Why to the How and Back Again

Mina Silberberg, PhD

ABOUT THE AUTHORS

Mina Silberberg is a faculty member in the Division of Community Health, Department of Family Medicine and Community Health, at Duke School of Medicine. She is also affiliated with the department's Division of Family Medicine, the Duke Global Health Institute, the Duke Margolis Institute for Health Policy, the Duke Department of Head and Neck Surgery & Communication Sciences, and the Duke Clinical and Translational Science Institute, where she serves as faculty director of the Community Engaged Research Initiative.

See also Callahan et al., p. 619.

In recent years, there has been remarkable growth in support for integrating social and medical care in the United States. Integration is primarily understood as screening in the health care setting for unmet social needs (e.g., housing, food, transportation, assistance with domestic violence) and referring patients to organizations that provide assistance in these areas. Other approaches to integration involve coverage of a portion of social care costs by third-party payers, as in current Medicaid waiver projects. The rationale for integration—the "why"—begins with the recognition that health is primarily driven by social conditions, termed "social determinants or drivers of health" (SDOH), and health disparities are primarily driven by differences in SDOH. Many observers anticipate that the growing prevalence of value-based health care (in which payment is based on outcomes rather than procedure volume) will lead to financial support for social care integration.

FROM THE WHY TO THE HOW

Our excitement over new approaches to improved health generally outstrips our attention to how we can successfully implement them, and social care integration is no exception. In this issue of *AJPH*, Callahan et al. (p. 619) tackle a portion of the "how" question for integration through a case study of Eskenazi Health, the safety net health care system serving Marion County, Indiana. Building off the National Academies of Science, Engineering, and Medicine report *Integrating Social Care Into the Delivery of Health Care: Moving Upstream to Improve the Nation's Health*,[1] they describe how Eskenazi developed the infrastructure to implement screening and referrals to social care, and they calculate the average annual expenditures associated with infrastructure development to be $2 360 000. Noting that Eskenazi's characteristics might in some ways result in lower-than-average costs (e.g., because of strong existing relationships with social care) and in other ways higher costs (e.g., because their patients have many social needs), they estimate that for most health care systems, integration infrastructure development costs will range from $1 million to $3 million annually for 5 to 10 years. (These are infrastructure development costs only, not taking into account, for example, additional funds needed to expand social care availability.)

In discussing their findings, Callahan et al. move further into the "how" of integration by asking who will pay the costs they have identified. They note that government and industry funding for social care tends to rely on short-term demonstration projects not conducive to developing durable infrastructure. Philanthropy sometimes offers longer-term investment, but competing for these funds means competing against the very organizations that address social needs.

So, how should we think about paying the costs of integration infrastructure development? In doing so, how should we use the kind of information provided by Callahan and his colleagues? One approach is to see such cost estimates as grist for an economic cost–benefit analysis to be undertaken by health care systems and payers to determine whether to make infrastructure investments. Certainly, if we are to think critically about the economic opportunity costs of social care integration, be realistic about its feasibility, and determine how it can be funded, we must explore integration's economic costs and cost savings. These considerations, however, should be part of a larger discussion. Cost–benefit analysis offers the allure of "technocratic" solutions to

AJPH June 2024, Vol. 114, No. 6

complex decisions; however, it elides critical questions about how we monetize nonfinancial costs and benefits, how we think about costs and benefits we cannot monetize, to whom costs and benefits accrue, short-term versus long-term impacts, and the complexity of cause and effect in the real world.[2]

A number of issues illustrate the importance of developing an analytic framework for integration decisions that moves beyond the financial concerns of health care providers and payers to a larger set of societal considerations. These issues make it clear that to think about the "how" of integration, we must rethink the "why" of integration—what we believe integration accomplishes and how we regard those results.

FROM THE HOW TO THE WHY

Callahan et al. point us in this direction when they highlight nonfinancial challenges of integration infrastructure development. They indicate the importance of building community resources, rather than supplanting them. They also cite concerns over the medicalization of social needs. There is, in fact, a tension between the concern over medicalization and expansion of the role of third-party payers,[3] which they cite as a piece of the funding solution. This tension does not negate the role of health care payers, but does highlight the importance of considering a variety of issues when thinking about how to support integration.

The importance of nonfinancial considerations in our approach to social care integration has been highlighted by Berkowitz et al.[4] They point out that addressing social needs sometimes improves health without reducing costs, particularly short-term costs. Moreover, this is also true of many clinical interventions that we nonetheless provide because they align with our values around health. The authors suggest that we treat social care the same way—thinking about our collective values, not just economic "value."

Berkowitz et al. also note that, to make financial benefits outweigh financial costs, some systems focus social care on those whose unmet social needs are linked to large health care expenditures. They question the alignment with our values of "equating deservingness of intervention with the likelihood of generating high healthcare costs" and caution against over-reliance on "market-oriented justifications" (i.e., cost savings to specific actors) for providing services.[4(p1917)] Similarly, I would argue, the logic of purely market-oriented justifications is challenged by the differential impact of such reasoning on different health care systems. For example, does the "deservingness" of patients with social care needs vary based on differences in the opportunity costs of integration for their health care providers?

Our analytic framework must also be based on a more complete understanding of the effects of social care integration than that which now dominates our discourse. Gottlieb et al. note that even when referrals for social needs do not result in those needs being met, patient health often improves.[5] Research suggests that the navigation services, strengthened patient connections to ambulatory care, and changes to health care delivery teams resulting from integration can enhance health by improving emotional support, ambulatory care use, and disease self-management. This broadened understanding of the "logic" behind social care screening and referrals changes the calculus around the benefits of incorporating social workers and community health workers into the clinical setting.

Moreover, in thinking about cause and effect, society must take the long view, although individual actors generally do not. Based on what we know of the effects of childhood environment,[6] for example, meeting housing, food, transportation, and personal safety needs can have a significant impact on the well-being and health of future generations; this impact will not be measured by short-term research. Callahan et al. have provided us with important information about the "how" of integration that can help inform deliberation and decision-making processes. Ideally these processes will take a broad societal perspective in assessing and considering the requirements and results of social integration, the value it provides, and the ways in which it aligns with our values. AJPH

CORRESPONDENCE

All correspondence should be directed to Mina Silberberg, Duke Division of Community Health, DUMC 104652, Durham, NC 27710 (e-mail: mina.silberberg@duke.edu). Reprints can be ordered at https://ajph.org by clicking the "Reprints" link.

PUBLICATION INFORMATION

Full Citation: Silberberg M. Integrating social care and medical care: from the why to the how and back again. *Am J Public Health*. 2024;114(6):543–545.

Acceptance Date: March 10, 2024.

DOI: https://doi.org/10.2105/AJPH.2024.307664

ACKNOWLEDGMENTS

The author thanks Kerry L. Haynie, PhD, for his review of and thoughts on this article.

CONFLICTS OF INTEREST

The author has no conflicts of interest to disclose.

REFERENCES

1. National Academies of Sciences, Engineering, and Medicine, Committee on Integrating Social Needs Care Into the Delivery of Health Care to Improve the Nation's Health. *Integrating Social Care Into the Delivery of Health Care: Moving Upstream to Improve the Nation's Health*. Washington, DC: National Academies Press; 2019.

2. Brown LD, Gusmano M. Introduction: evaluation in analytic theory and political practice. *J Health Polit Policy Law.* 2013;38(6):1071–1079. https://doi.org/10.1215/03616878-2373139
3. Wilkins C. Connecting permanent supportive housing to health care delivery and payment systems: opportunities and challenges. *Am J Psychiatr Rehabil.* 2015;18(1):65–86. https://doi.org/10.1080/15487768.2015.1001690
4. Berkowitz SA, Baggett TP, Edwards ST. Addressing health-related social needs: value-based care or values-based care? *J Gen Intern Med.* 2019;34(9):1916–1918. https://doi.org/10.1007/s11606-019-05087-3
5. Gottlieb LM, Hessler D, Wing H, Gonzalez-Rocha A, Cartier Y, Fichtenberg C. Revising the logic model behind health care's social care investments. *Milbank Q.* 2024; epub ahead of print January 25, 2024. https://doi.org/10.1111/1468-0009.12690
6. Morelli V. Social determinants of health: an overview for the primary care provider. *Prim Care.* 2023;50(4):507–525. https://doi.org/10.1016/j.pop.2023.04.004

Building Momentum for a Safe System Approach to Reduce Road Traffic Injuries in the United States

Johnathon P. Ehsani, PhD, MPH, Glendedora Dolce, MPH, and Jeffrey P. Michael, EdD

ABOUT THE AUTHORS

All authors are with the Department of Health Policy and Management, Johns Hopkins Bloomberg School of Public Health, Baltimore, MD.

See also Dragan and Glied, p. 633.

AJPH June 2024, Vol. 114, No. 6

Roadway designs have an effect on how people drive. Designs that prioritize the flow of cars often do so at the expense of safety for those who are walking and biking.[1] Dangerous designs are more likely to be located in low-income neighborhoods, leading to disparities in road traffic injuries. As a result, communities of color experience higher crash death rates than those in predominantly White areas, and low-income neighborhoods have fatality rates that are three to four times higher than those in wealthier areas.[2]

Vision Zero or Safe System interventions can address these disparities. In 2014, New York City was one of the first US jurisdictions to introduce a comprehensive range of policies termed Vision Zero.[3] Vision Zero is so called because of the commitment to no deaths from road traffic crashes and was inspired by the Safe Systems approach pioneered in Sweden and the Netherlands in the 1990s. In the Safe System approach, the focus shifts from "How can people use the transportation system more safely?" to "How can the system be made safe for people to use?" The Safe System implementation in the United States gained momentum owing to the 2021 Bipartisan Infrastructure Law, which introduced a new Safe Streets and Roads for All grant program. This program provides $5 billion over five years to support local improvements that align with Safe System principles.[4] The US Department of Transportation followed this with the first national roadway safety strategy based on the Safe System approach.[5]

The study by Dragan and Glied (p. 633) in this issue of *AJPH* notably highlights three important aspects of Vision Zero programs. First, Vision Zero is designed to enhance the safety of all road users, rather than targeting vehicle occupants only. Consequently, it led to a dramatic reduction in road traffic injuries among the most disadvantaged groups. Second, Vision Zero policies are scalable and sustainable.[6] Most interventions included in the program involve changes to the infrastructure and roadway environment that are "self-enforcing" rather than requiring continual policing for effectiveness.[7] Third, because they used Medicaid data, the authors were able to quantify the cost savings resulting from Vision Zero policies, which is one of the first times that health benefits have been quantified in the US context.

Dragan and Glied's findings are particularly encouraging because the Safe System approach is intended to improve both safety and equity. Using Medicaid claims data from New York City and surrounding counties, they demonstrated that Vision Zero policies disproportionately benefited low-income and Black residents in terms of road traffic injuries. The central goal of a Safe System is zero traffic deaths and serious injuries, and this demands investment according to need. Communities that have previously suffered from underinvestment will necessarily require more resources to reach zero traffic deaths than communities where safety improvements have already been made. Because Safe Systems cannot be implemented everywhere at once, areas most in need can be prioritized.[7]

The Safe System approach demands a careful analysis of safety issues and identification of root causes. For instance, intersection crashes, which contribute to approximately one quarter of fatalities and about half of all injuries, prove lethal because of the vulnerability of conventional intersection layouts to common human errors such as distraction and inattention. These errors often result in high-speed side-impact collisions that exceed human injury tolerance thresholds. In the Safe System framework, high-risk intersections are replaced by roundabouts, which reduce speeds and alter vehicle trajectories to lessen the impact of typical driver errors such as failure to notice traffic signals, oncoming vehicles, or pedestrians. Roundabouts are engineered to require drivers to decelerate and align with the flow of traffic, thereby reducing the likelihood of severe injuries by preventing deadly high-speed head-on and side-impact collisions.

As mentioned previously, roundabouts and other strategies in the Safe System framework are engineered to be self-enforcing. These designs incorporate physical elements such as narrowed lanes, speed humps, tighter corner-turning radii, and chicanes to guide drivers toward safe speeds, rather than relying solely on posted speed limits. Roads are planned so that the comfortable driving pace aligns with the safe speed. Additionally, features such as separated bike lanes and intersections equipped with clearly marked crosswalks, raised medians, and pedestrian refuge islands serve to decelerate traffic and ensure that pedestrians and cyclists remain visible to drivers. By reducing speeds, reaction times are increased, making crashes less probable and mitigating the severity of any conflicts that do occur. Implementation of the Safe System approach entails a dedication to proactive safety enhancements, introducing them preemptively in all areas prone to crashes, rather than delaying action until injuries occur. This approach emphasizes prevention over reaction to reduce crashes and can be adapted to communities of diverse sizes and demographics.

A question that naturally arises is why the United States has only recently adopted Safe System approaches? One reason is the entrenched institutional resistance to large-scale change. Existing road design standards and practice guidelines are codified in manuals and protocols, whereas most funding channels have incentivized traditional practices rather than adopting a Safe System approach. Although institutional inertia does not justify maintaining the status quo, overcoming it will demand concerted efforts. Another obstacle that must be overcome in the United States is the need to rectify past and present disparities in transportation system investments. Although the Safe System approach holds promise for addressing historical injustices in transportation, implementing this approach necessitates sensitivity and a steadfast commitment to inclusive planning processes that genuinely engage communities.

The United States is still in the early stages of adoption of the Safe System approach. Despite political support, a relatively modest number of jurisdictions have adopted the comprehensive set of strategies that New York City implemented as part of Vision Zero. The article by Dragan and Glied adds much needed momentum to the movement in this country. Jurisdictions considering Vision Zero policies should proceed with optimism that implementation will advance both safety and equity. AJPH

CORRESPONDENCE

Correspondence should be sent to Johnathon P. Ehsani, PhD, Department of Health Policy and Management, Johns Hopkins Bloomberg School of Public Health, 624 N. Broadway, Hampton House 555, Baltimore, MD 21205 (e-mail: johnathon.ehsani@jhu.edu). Reprints can be ordered at http://www.ajph.org by clicking the "Reprints" link.

PUBLICATION INFORMATION

Full Citation: Ehsani JP, Dolce G, Michael JP. Building momentum for a Safe System approach to reduce road traffic injuries in the United States. *Am J Public Health*. 2024;114(6):546–547.

Acceptance Date: March 25, 2024.

DOI: https://doi.org/10.2105/AJPH.2024.307674

ORCID iD:

Johnathon P. Ehsani https://orcid.org/0000-0001-9869-1679

CONTRIBUTORS

J. P. Ehsani and G. Dolce drafted the original version of the editorial, and J. P. Michael revised it.

CONFLICTS OF INTEREST

The authors have no conflicts of interest to declare.

REFERENCES

1. Michael JP, Wells NM, Shahum L, Bidigare-Curtis HN, Greenberg SF, Xu T. Roadway safety, design & equity: a paradigm shift. *J Transp Health*. 2021; 23:101260. https://doi.org/10.1016/j.jth.2021.101260
2. Marshall WE, Ferenchak NN. Assessing equity and urban/rural road safety disparities in the US. *J Urban*. 2017;10(4):422–441. https://doi.org/10.1080/17549175.2017.1310748
3. US Department of Transportation. Vision Zero in New York City. Available at: https://safety.fhwa.dot.gov/zerodeaths/vz_nyc. Accessed March 6, 2024.
4. US Department of Transportation. Safe Streets and Roads for All (SS4A) grant program. Available at: https://www.transportation.gov/grants/SS4A. Accessed August 4, 2023.
5. US Department of Transportation. USDOT national roadway safety strategy. 2022. Available at: https://www.transportation.gov/nrss/usdot-national-roadway-safety-strategy. Accessed March 27, 2023.
6. Welle B, Sharpin AB, Adriazola-Steil C, et al. Sustainable and safe: a vision and guidance for zero road deaths. January 11, 2018. Available at: https://www.wri.org/research/sustainable-and-safe-vision-and-guidance-zero-road-deaths. Accessed April 6, 2024.
7. Ehsani JP, Michael JP, MacKenzie EJ. The future of road safety: challenges and opportunities. *Milbank Q*. 2023;101(suppl 1):613–636. https://doi.org/10.1111/1468-0009.12644

Housing Ends Homelessness

Joshua D. Bamberger, MD, MPH

ABOUT THE AUTHOR

Joshua D. Bamberger is a clinical professor in the Department of Family and Community Medicine at the University of California San Francisco and is a primary care physician with the San Francisco Department of Public Health and the Medical Service of the San Francisco Veterans Affairs Health Care System.

See also Wilkinson et al., p. 610.

According to the annual Point in Time Count, the number of veterans experiencing homelessness in the United States has declined by more than 50% since 2010. Over that same period in the United States, there has been an increase in the total number of adults experiencing homelessness.[1]

Housing ends homelessness. While the prevalence of mental illness and substance use is higher among people who experience homelessness than in the general population, housing will always be the foundation necessary to end the homelessness epidemic in the United States.

REDUCTIONS IN VETERAN HOMELESSNESS

At present, 12 communities across the United States have effectively and sustainably ended homelessness for veterans.[2] Since 2008, more than 144 000 veterans have been assisted into permanent housing with the help of our nation's most effective program to reduce and end homelessness, the Housing and Urban Development VA Supportive Housing (HUD VASH) program.[3] HUD VASH provides the funding to bridge the gap between what a veteran can contribute in rent and the market rate rent in a community. In addition, the VA is our nation's largest single-payer health care system and provides care and treatment of veterans who suffer from the chronic medical and behavioral health conditions that can lead to or result from living on the streets.

While a combination of state, federal, and local programs make similar investments in permanent housing in some communities, no other subpopulation has seen such progress in reducing and ending homelessness. One reason why there has been such progress among veterans in the United States is that in addition to robust funding for permanent housing, the VA has also funded Supportive Services for Veteran Families (SSVF), a veteran-centric program that provides flexible funding to overcome the myriad impediments that get in the way of helping individuals and families move from homelessness to housing or to prevent homelessness in the first place.

In this issue of *AJPH*, Wilkinson et al. (p. 610) provide an overview of the first 10 years of SSVF and describe how it has been an essential component of improved outcomes for veterans experiencing homelessness. Funding for SSVF successfully escapes the constraints of the heavily bureaucratic VA system of care by pushing funding out to community-based organizations. Over the 10 years of its existence, SSVF has grown dramatically and been used for an array of services from assisting people to reunite with loved ones in their community to paying for rental gaps that could lead to homelessness and even sometimes paying for car repairs so veterans can get to the appointments necessary to get a job or get a home. No other federal program for people experiencing homelessness is similarly structured, and few local or state programs provide funding that incorporates the flexibility and scale of SSVF. In addition to SSVF and HUD VASH, the VA also funds the Grant and Per Diem Programs that offer residential substance use treatment and rapidly accessible, noncongregate, short-term housing to keep veterans safe and quickly move them off the street while they work with the VA and community-based organizations to obtain permanent housing. These three lines of business within the VA are the cornerstones that have most likely led to the impressive progress in reducing homelessness among veterans.

MORE THAT CAN BE DONE TO HELP END VETERAN HOMELESSNESS

Despite considerable success, more could be done. It is possible that a more flexible program than SSVF such as providing a basic income to veterans experiencing homelessness could be even more effective and simpler to administer than SSVF.[4] In Los Angeles, California, local housing authorities have issued more than 2500 HUD VASH vouchers that are sitting unused by veterans[5] while more than 4000 veterans in Los Angeles County experience homelessness.[6] Inadequate numbers of outreach staff contribute to a system-wide failure to identify the housing needs of homeless veterans while SSVF has struggled to be used to pay for essential housing locator functions to identify landlords who have vacant units and are willing to rent to veterans. The inability to successfully use already allocated funding for HUD VASH is common across many high-rent, low-vacancy communities. Because SSVF must be issued to an individual veteran, there are significant administrative barriers that prevent a master-leasing strategy that could support set-aside blocks of units for veterans to live stably with other veterans.

The VA has been slow to establish a diversity of medical services (such as embedding full-time nurses in housing) across project-based housing programs so that veterans with complex medical and behavioral health needs can be matched with housing with on-site services that meet their needs. This can lead to unnecessary use of high-cost inpatient stays within the VA hospital system. Lastly, the VA has no line of business similar to Medicaid Assisted Living Waivers[7] that can provide funding for residential care facilities to serve the small but growing subset of veterans with needs too medically complex for independent housing but who do not need or qualify for the institutional-based care of a skilled nursing facility. These unfortunate veterans often cycle between very expensive hospital-based care and inadequate shelter or independent housing until they become sick enough to develop a skilled nursing need. The demand for a program that supports assisted living facilities for veterans will only increase over the next decade as the expected number of homeless veterans aged older than 60 years also increases dramatically.[8]

CONCLUSIONS

Having provided primary care for the past 35 years for adults experiencing homelessness and primary care for veterans for the past 10 years, I see little difference in the clinical presentation between the veterans I serve in the VA and the nonveterans I serve in the general public health system. However, for my patients who happen to have served in the military, their time experiencing homelessness is usually rare, brief, and nonrecurring. Ending homelessness for an individual outside of the VA system of care is sometimes possible but is much more complicated and unpredictable. I have often wondered what it would be like to provide care for adults experiencing homelessness in Northern European countries that have universal health care, truly embrace Housing First,[9] and provide adequate funding for affordable housing.[10] While the fractured US health care and housing systems have a long way to go to deliver the housing outcomes seen in Europe, what the VA has developed over these past 20 years gets us closer than any other system in the United States. SSVF fills in the gaps in the system and is catalytic in leading to this success. For that, we should all be proud of what this country can do while it serves as a road map of what we have yet to achieve. AJPH

CORRESPONDENCE

Correspondence should be sent to Joshua D. Bamberger, Downtown VA Clinic, 401 3rd St, San Francisco, CA 94107 (e-mail: joshua.bamberger@ucsf.edu). Reprints can be ordered at https://ajph.org by clicking the "Reprints" link.

PUBLICATION INFORMATION

Full Citation: Bamberger JD. Housing ends homelessness. *Am J Public Health*. 2024;114(6):548–549.

Acceptance Date: March 24, 2024.

DOI: https://doi.org/10.2105/AJPH.2024.307671

CONFLICTS OF INTEREST

The author reports no conflicts of interest.

REFERENCES

1. National Alliance to End Homelessness. State of homelessness: 2023 edition. January 6, 2024. Available at: https://endhomelessness.org/homelessness-in-america/homelessness-statistics/state-of-homelessness. Accessed February 15, 2024.
2. Community Solutions. Functional zero. March 26, 2024. Available at: https://community.solutions/built-for-zero/functional-zero. Accessed March 26, 2024.
3. Center for Evidence-based Solutions to Homelessness. HUD-VASH vouchers. Available at: http://www.evidenceonhomelessness.com/factsheet/hud-vash-vouchers. Accessed February 15, 2024.
4. Henwood BF, Kim BKE, Stein A, et al. Miracle Friends and Miracle Money in California: a mixed-methods experiment of social support and guaranteed income for people experiencing homelessness. Research Square. Published online September 6, 2023. https://doi.org/10.21203/rs.3.rs-3287846/v1
5. Veterans Affairs Greater Los Angeles Healthcare System Master Plan. GLA's homeless programs: Community Engagement & Reintegration Service (CERS). Available at: https://westlamasterplan.org/p/CERS. Accessed February 15, 2024.
6. Los Angeles Homeless Services Authority. Homeless count. 2023. Available at: https://www.lahsa.org/data-refresh. Accessed February 15, 2024.
7. Cameron J. What is a Medicaid waiver? Your guide to Medicaid home and community-based services. AssistedLiving.org. November 3, 2023. Available at: https://www.assistedliving.org/what-is-a-medicaid-waiver. Accessed February 15, 2024.
8. Culhane DP, Metraux S, Byrne T, Stino M, Bainbridge J. The age structure of contemporary homelessness: evidence and implications for public policy. *Anal Soc Issues Public Policy*. 2013;13(1):228–244. https://doi.org/10.1111/asap.12004
9. US Department of Housing and Urban Development. Housing First in permanent supportive housing. Available at: https://files.hudexchange.info/resources/documents/Housing-First-Permanent-Supportive-Housing-Brief.pdf. Accessed February 15, 2024.
10. US Department of Housing and Urban Development. Two essays on unequal growth in housing. *Cityscape*. 2020;22(2). Available at: https://www.huduser.gov/portal/periodicals/cityscpe/vol22num2/article4.html. Accessed February 15, 2024.

Cannabis and Alcohol Involvement in Motor Vehicle Crashes: Reflections in the Era of Legalization

Mark Asbridge, PhD, and Jeff Brubacher, MD

ABOUT THE AUTHORS

Mark Asbridge is with the Department of Community Health and Epidemiology, Dalhousie University, Halifax, Nova Scotia, Canada. Jeff Brubacher is with the Department of Emergency Medicine, Faculty of Medicine, University of British Columbia, Vancouver, BC, Canada.

AJPH June 2024, Vol. 114, No. 6

An article by Lira et al.,[1] published in 2021, examined trends in cannabis involvement and risk of alcohol coinvolvement in motor vehicle fatalities over an 18-year period in the United States. Considerable attention has been directed to this work and is reflective of our growing interest in the issue of recreational cannabis use and its potential impacts on driving ability, road safety, and public health. A review of publication trends indicates a substantial increase in research studies on cannabis use and driving since 2015. Research has examined changing prevalence rates in youth and adult populations, crash risk, social and economic costs, risk perceptions, standardized testing, enforcement, interventions, and policy approaches. The work of Lira et al. was an important contribution to this rapidly growing body of work.

THE CHANGING RATE OF CRASHES INVOLVING CANNABIS

This study resonated with the public health community as it drew attention to several important trends in the context of impaired driving research and road safety. First, the rate of cannabis-involved fatal collisions, drawing on data from the Fatality Analysis Reporting System, has increased substantially from 9.0% of fatal crashes in 2000 to 21.5% in 2018.[1] The greater-than-twofold increase in presence of cannabis in fatal motor vehicle crashes observed by Lira et al. is not unique to the United States and has also been noted in studies of nonfatal crash–involved drivers and non–crash-involved drivers in other jurisdictions.[2–4]

The important question posed by Lira et al. is, why are we witnessing a rise in cannabis-involved fatal crashes? The authors suggest that the rise "could be attributable to shifting cannabis policies enabling expansion of medical and recreational cannabis markets, changing societal attitudes toward cannabis, and other factors such as increased cannabis potency."[1(p1982)] There is certainly a case to be made for the first two arguments. The last 15 to 20 years have witnessed a considerable shift in both the formal and informal regulation of cannabis consumption across North America and in other parts of the globe. This includes the broader normalization of recreational cannabis consumption such that consumption is generally tolerated or even accepted irrespective of the presence of policies decriminalizing or legalizing recreational cannabis use.[5] This can be coupled with formal policy responses that have expanded the scope of medical cannabis consumption or have legalized recreational cannabis use. In North America, Canada (2018), Mexico (2021), and 24 states and the District of Columbia in the United States have legalized recreational cannabis consumption, and recreational cannabis sales are legal in Canada and in 22 US states. Early evidence from some of those jurisdictions shows significant increases in the presence of cannabis in injured drivers as well as in non–crash-involved drivers following the legalization of recreational cannabis use[6,7]; however, not all studies have observed significant changes in rates of driving after cannabis use or related activities following legalization.[8,9]

THE COINVOLVEMENT OF CANNABIS AND ALCOHOL

Second, the work of Lira et al. points to the concerning interplay between the presence of cannabis and alcohol in fatal crashes, where cannabis was strongly associated with alcohol coinvolvement across differing blood alcohol concentration (BAC) levels (0.01%–0.049%; 0.05% to 0.079%; and 0.08% and higher). Population survey data show similar trends: 14% of respondents who admitted to driving within two hours of smoking cannabis or within four hours of consuming edible cannabis products also reported they had driven under the influence of cannabis and alcohol in combination within the past 30 days.[10] The coinvolvement of alcohol and cannabis in fatally injured drivers represents a concerning trend given public health gains in the reduction of alcohol-impaired driving observed over the past 25 years. For example, population surveys, roadside surveys, and hospital and coroner data have noted substantial declines in drinking and driving behaviors, particularly among drivers aged younger than 25 years, as well as the observation that rates of driving under the influence of alcohol have dropped below rates for driving after using cannabis in certain populations.[11,12]

More importantly, this work speaks to the potential interaction of alcohol and cannabis and how concurrent use of cannabis and alcohol affect driving performance, crash risk, and road safety. A more limited body of research has examined the combined use of alcohol and cannabis on driving performance and crash risk, and the exact nature of this relationship is difficult to assess. While both have an impairing effect on driving, the impact of their interaction is complicated. Cannabis is typically associated with poorer reaction time, lane violations, and slower driving speeds, while alcohol is associated with increased speed and more reckless driving actions.[13] The level of impairment when alcohol and cannabis are combined is also questioned: some studies suggest the effect is multiplicative, whereby the combined effect is stronger than what would be expected from simply adding the effect of cannabis and alcohol to crash risk, while others suggest the effect is additive[14]; there is also some evidence that lower-dose-tetrahydrocannabinol (THC) cannabis might mitigate select dangerous driving actions associated with alcohol such as speeding.[15] Despite this heterogeneity, the consistent observation is that the combined use of cannabis and alcohol imposes greater deficits on driving performance and an increased crash risk relative to the use of either substance alone.[14]

IMPLICATIONS ON POLICY, PRACTICE, AND RESEARCH

As articulated by Lira et al., further research is warranted to better understand how differing levels of cannabis consumption, as well as distinct kinds of cannabinoids, interact with alcohol consumption to affect driving ability and road safety. Recent studies have begun this endeavor by examining the driving tasks most affected by the concurrent use of cannabis and alcohol relative to the use of either substance alone. For example, the combined use of cannabis and alcohol produces greater deficits in lateral control, lateral position variability, and reaction time than either alcohol or cannabis alone.[14] Other work has looked at how the mode of cannabis consumption, alone and when used with alcohol, affects driving performance. Equally important questions include "At what consumption level does the concurrent use of alcohol and cannabis begin to affect driving ability?" and "Does cannabis interfere with established protective associations between alcohol policies and drinking and driving crashes?" These are all important areas for future research.

The interplay between cannabis and alcohol is also highly relevant to health policy and criminal law. As Lira et al. noted, "Adopting a lower permissible BAC threshold for those with cannabis in their system may be a policy strategy to reduce [motor vehicle crash] harms from concurrent and simultaneous use of alcohol and cannabis."[1(p1983)] This is, in fact, what some jurisdictions have done through the introduction of specific penalties for driving when both cannabis and alcohol are present. For example, in Canada, it is a potentially indictable offense (similar to a felony in the United States) to drive a vehicle with blood THC of greater than or equal to 5 nanograms per milliliter or with blood alcohol greater than or equal to 80 milligrams per deciliter, whereas when both alcohol and cannabis are present the legal limits are lowered and it is a potentially indictable offense to drive with blood THC of greater than or equal to 2.5 nanograms per milliliter and blood alcohol greater than or equal to 50 milligrams per deciliter. Similar policies in other jurisdictions are likely to emerge with the ongoing expansion of cannabis legalization.

Moving forward, it is important that evidence continues to be collected to assess trends in cannabis-involved driving, either alone or concurrently with alcohol, and its impact on crash rates and road safety. The urgency of this work is predicated on the ongoing liberalization of recreational cannabis consumption globally. This requires roadside and population surveys to examine prevalence in the general driving population and studies of injured drivers to assess prevalence in crash-involved drivers. Well-designed case—control studies are needed to optimally examine the crash risk of cannabis (at different THC levels) both alone and in combination with alcohol. Experimental studies are necessary to further investigate the effect of cannabis, both alone and together with alcohol, on the specific tasks required for safe driving. In addition, improved methods to screen drivers under the influence of cannabis, particularly at the roadside, are essential to facilitate more effective approaches for detection, enforcement, and prevention. Finally, primary research must be coupled with continuing policy development and evaluation to maximize road safety efforts. AJPH

CORRESPONDENCE

Correspondence should be sent to Mark Asbridge, Department of Community Health and Epidemiology, Dalhousie University, Centre for Clinical Research, 5790 University Ave, Halifax, Nova Scotia, Canada, B3H 1V7 (e-mail: mark.asbridge@dal.ca). Reprints can be ordered at https://ajph.org by clicking the "Reprints" link.

PUBLICATION INFORMATION

Full Citation: Asbridge M, Brubacher J. Cannabis and alcohol involvement in motor vehicle crashes: reflections in the era of legalization. *Am J Public Health*. 2024;114(6):550–552.

Acceptance Date: March 5, 2024.

DOI: https://doi.org/10.2105/AJPH.2024.307657

CONTRIBUTORS

M. Asbridge and J. Brubacher contributed to the conceptualization, drafting, and revision of the article, and approved the final version.

CONFLICTS OF INTEREST

The authors have no conflicts of interest to declare.

REFERENCES

1. Lira MC, Heeren TC, Buczek M, et al. Trends in cannabis involvement and risk of alcohol involvement in motor vehicle crash fatalities in the United States, 2000–2018. *Am J Public Health*. 2021;111(11):1976–1985. https://doi.org/10.2105/AJPH.2021.306466
2. Robertson RD, Hing MM, Pashley CR, Brown SW, Vanlaar WG. Prevalence and trends of drugged driving in Canada. *Accid Anal Prev*. 2017;99(pt A):236–241. https://doi.org/10.1016/j.aap.2016.12.008
3. Davey JD, Armstrong KA, Freeman JE, Parkes A. Alcohol and illicit substances associated with fatal crashes in Queensland: an examination of the 2011 to 2015 coroner's findings. *Forensic Sci Int*. 2020;312:110190. https://doi.org/10.1016/j.forsciint.2020.110190
4. Brubacher JR, Chan H, Erdelyi S, et al. Cannabis use as a risk factor for causing motor vehicle crashes: a prospective study. *Addiction*. 2019;114(9):1616–1626. https://doi.org/10.1111/add.14663
5. Duff C, Asbridge M, Brochu S, et al. A Canadian perspective on cannabis normalization among adults. *Addict Res Theory*. 2012;20(4):271–283. https://doi.org/10.3109/16066359.2011.618957
6. Brubacher JR, Chan H, Erdelyi S, Staples JA, Asbridge M, Mann RE. Cannabis legalization and detection of tetrahydrocannabinol in injured drivers. *N Engl J Med*. 2022;386(2):148–156. https://doi.org/10.1056/NEJMsa2109371
7. Tolan NV, Krasowski MD, Mathias PC, et al. Cannabis positivity rates in 17 emergency departments across the United States with varying degrees of marijuana legalization. *Clin Toxicol (Phila)*. 2023;61(4):248–259. https://doi.org/10.1080/15563650.2023.2177552
8. Imtiaz S, Nigatu YT, Ali F, et al. Cannabis legalization and driving under the influence of cannabis and driving under the influence of alcohol among adult and adolescent drivers in Ontario, Canada (2001–2019). *Drug Alcohol Depend*. 2024;255;111060. https://doi.org/10.1016/j.drugalcdep.2023.111060.
9. Callaghan RC, Sanches M, Vander Heiden J, et al. Canada's cannabis legalization and drivers' traffic-injury presentations to emergency departments in Ontario and Alberta, 2015–2019. *Drug Alcohol Depend*. 2021;228:109008. https://doi.org/10.1016/j.drugalcdep.2021.109008
10. Government of Canada. Canadian Cannabis Survey 2022: Summary. Available at: https://www.canada.ca/en/health-canada/services/drugs-medication/cannabis/research-data/canadian-cannabis-survey-2022-summary.html. Accessed December 14, 2023.
11. Beirness DJ, Beasley EE, McClafferty K. *Alcohol and Drug Use Among Drivers in Ontario: Findings From the 2017 Roadside Survey*. Ministry of Transportation; 2017.
12. Beirness DJ, Gu KW, Lowe NJ, et al. Cannabis, alcohol and other drug findings in fatally injured drivers in Ontario. *Traffic Inj Prev*. 2021;22(1):1–6. https://doi.org/10.1080/15389588.2020.1847281
13. Ronen A, Chassidim HS, Gershon P, et al. The effect of alcohol, THC and their combination on perceived effects, willingness to drive and performance of driving and non-driving tasks. *Accid Anal Prev*. 2010;42(6):1855–1865. https://doi.org/10.1016/j.aap.2010.05.006
14. Simmons SM, Caird JK, Sterzer F, Asbridge M. The effects of cannabis and alcohol on driving performance and driver behaviour: a systematic review and meta-analysis. *Addiction*. 2022;117(7):1843–1856. https://doi.org/10.1111/add.15770
15. Hartman RL, Brown TL, Milavetz G, et al. Cannabis effects on driving lateral control with and without alcohol. *Drug Alcohol Depend*. 2015;154:25–37. https://doi.org/10.1016/j.drugalcdep.2015.06.015

Disparities in Overdose Deaths: Looking Back at Larochelle and Colleagues' 2021 Paper

Nora D. Volkow, MD, Beth Han, PhD, MD, MPH, and Redonna K. Chandler, PhD

ABOUT THE AUTHORS

All authors are with the National Institute on Drug Abuse, National Institutes of Health, Bethesda, MD.

In the Healing Community Study (HCS), we aimed to show that implementation of a battery of evidence-based interventions to expand (1) access to naloxone, (2) the number of patients treated with medications for opioid use disorder (OUD), and (3) safer opioid prescribing practices would result in a 40% reduction of overdose deaths.[1] In the HCS, we selected 67 rural and urban communities from four states (Kentucky, Ohio, Massachusetts, and New York), which at the time had some of the highest overdose rates in the country. We randomized communities either to receive the HCS intervention for 18 months or to serve as a control (wave 1), followed by implementation of the HCS intervention for the subsequent 18 months in the control communities (wave 2).[2]

Communities in partnership with academicians selected the evidence-based interventions and implemented them in collaboration with the health care, behavioral health, and justice systems, as well as state agencies, while monitoring progress using data indicators. This first step required that the communities obtain baseline data on demographics, overdose mortality, treatment capabilities, community support organizations, and other resources.[3]

The article by Larochelle et al.[4] is based on the baseline data from the four states that were part of the HCS. Larochelle et al. reported that from 2018 to 2019, the overdose deaths appeared to have stabilized except among non-Hispanic Black individuals (hereafter Black individuals), for whom overdose deaths increased by nearly 40%. We did not know then that the period of stabilization observed during 2018 to 2019 (except for Black individuals) would be so short-lived, nor did we imagine that four years later the overdose deaths would increase 53% from 70 630 in 2019[5] to 108 212 in 2022.[6] Larochelle et al. corroborated and brought attention to the marked increases in overdose mortality among Black individuals,[4] which continued to contribute to the unprecedented rise in overdose mortality in the subsequent years.[7,8]

Initially, the opioid overdose crisis most heavily affected non-Hispanic White people primarily because of overprescribing prescription opioid medications. Around 2010 to 2011, the demographics started to shift, coinciding first with a rise in heroin overdoses and subsequently a steep rise in overdoses from illicit fentanyl and its analogs.[9] By 2019, it was well established that the main driver of overdose deaths was fentanyl, which accounted for 73% (36 359 of 49 860) of opioid overdose deaths that year.[5]

However, it was difficult to predict how rapidly fentanyl would take over the illicit drug market across the United States and contaminate the drug supply, including that of heroin, stimulant drugs, and counterfeit pills. This shift in the drug supply exposed individuals who did not use opioids, and hence had no tolerance to them, to overdoses when they consumed contaminated products. Even for people with histories of heroin use, the much greater potency of fentanyl increased overdose risk. Contamination of cocaine and heroin used by Black individuals, coupled with racial/ethnic inequity in opioid prevention, intervention, and treatment resources, likely contributed to the rise in overdose mortality first noted in 2018.[7]

Another major event that could not have been predicted at the time the Larochelle et al. article was written was the COVID-19 pandemic. The pandemic disrupted the lives of communities and was exacerbated among people who use drugs, including those with an OUD. The COVID-19 pandemic affected all demographics but was particularly catastrophic among racial/ethnic minority groups, most notably Black individuals and Hispanics. From the beginning, clear disparities emerged in COVID-19–related morbidity and mortality for communities of color. These communities were at higher risk of infection owing to hazardous labor–related exposures, living conditions, or incarceration and had worse outcomes because of inadequate access to quality health care and higher rates of comorbidities.[10] Meanwhile, isolation, death of loved ones, loss of jobs, erosion of community support, and rise in homelessness affected individuals of racial/ethnic minority groups especially hard, increasing substance use and relapse for those with substance use disorders, including OUD.

Drug overdose mortality increased 45% over the first years of the pandemic.[11] As was the case for COVID-19–related morbidity and mortality, overdose mortality disproportionally affected racial/ethnic minority groups, notably Black individuals and non-Hispanic American Indian and Alaska Native persons. Among Black individuals, the overdose mortality rate per 100 000 rose from 17.1 in 2016 to 24.8 in 2019[5]; then it rose to 47.7 in 2022: a 179% increase from 2016.[6] In 2022, non-Hispanic American Indian and Alaska Native people, who were not part of the HCS communities, had the highest overdose mortality rate (64.4 per 100 000)[6] across racial/ethnic groups.

The COVID-19 pandemic facilitated changes in the provision of medications for OUD, lowering the requirements for take-home methadone by opioid treatment programs and facilitating the initiation of buprenorphine via telehealth, including from out-of-state providers. The use of telehealth to treat and manage substance use disorders and comorbidities was also accelerated. These changes proved to be lifesaving because they expanded the reach for treating OUD into rural areas, jails, prisons, and harm reduction programs. They increased the number of new initiates into buprenorphine treatment and helped improve retention in treatment during the challenging times of the COVID-19 pandemic.[12] Moreover, the findings that the changes in the provision of medications for OUD via telemedicine improved outcomes provided evidence to support their continuation after the termination of the COVID-19 emergency period.[12]

Since the Larochelle et al. article[4] was published, we have learned much both from the HCS and from how communities and providers addressed the challenges of taking care of people suffering from OUD amid the collision of two devastating crises: the COVID-19 pandemic and the overdose crisis (Box 1). The call by Larochelle et al. for targeted interventions to support Black communities was prescient and is as crucial now as it was then if we want to eliminate health inequities and successfully address the overdose crisis. AJPH

BOX 1— Additional Lessons Learned About the Need for Timely Data on Drug Use Patterns and Overdoses to Guide Interventions

Tailor interventions that are sensitive to demographics
Facilitate access to MOUD using diverse settings and models of care
Tackle polysubstance use and overdoses
Treat and support pregnant women with SUD, including OUD
Involve the community in sustaining OUD treatment and recovery
Target treatment of OUD among adolescents
Use prevention to avert overdoses, including among people with occasional misuse of illicitly manufactured prescription drugs

Note. MOUD = medications for opioid use disorder; OUD = opioid use disorder; SUD = substance use disorder.

CORRESPONDENCE

Correspondence should be sent to Nora D. Volkow, 3WFN Room 09D20, MSC 6025, 301 North Stonestreet Ave, Bethesda, MD 20892 (e-mail: nvolkow@nida.nih.gov). Reprints can be ordered at http://www.ajph.org by clicking the "Reprints" link.

PUBLICATION INFORMATION

Full Citation: Volkow ND, Han B, Chandler RK. Disparities in overdose deaths: looking back at Larochelle and colleagues' 2021 paper. *Am J Public Health.* 2024;114(6):553–555.

Acceptance Date: March 7, 2024.

DOI: https://doi.org/10.2105/AJPH.2024.307659

CONTRIBUTORS

N. D. Volkow conceptualized this project and drafted the editorial. All authors edited and finalized the editorial.

ACKNOWLEDGMENTS

We would like to thank the participating communities, participants, researchers, clinicians, and social service and harm reduction service providers of the Healing Community Study.

Note. The findings and conclusions of this study are those of the authors and do not necessarily reflect the views of the National Institute on Drug Abuse of the National Institutes of Health or the US Department of Health and Human Services.

CONFLICTS OF INTEREST

The authors have no conflicts of interest to disclose.

REFERENCES

1. Chandler RK, Villani J, Clarke T, McCance-Katz EF, Volkow ND. Addressing opioid overdose deaths: the vision for the HEALing communities study. *Drug Alcohol Depend.* 2020;217:108329. https://doi.org/10.1016/j.drugalcdep.2020.108329
2. HEALing Communities Study Consortium. The HEALing (Helping to End Addiction Long-term SM) Communities study: protocol for a cluster randomized trial at the community level to reduce opioid overdose deaths through implementation of an integrated set of evidence-based practices. *Drug Alcohol Depend.* 2020;217:108335. https://doi.org/10.1016/j.drugalcdep.2020.108335
3. Wu E, Villani J, Davis A, et al. Community dashboards to support data-informed decision-making in the HEALing Communities study. *Drug Alcohol Depend.* 2020;217:108331. https://doi.org/10.1016/j.drugalcdep.2020.108331
4. Larochelle MR, Slavova S, Root ED, et al. Disparities in opioid overdose death trends by race/ethnicity, 2018–2019, from the HEALing Communities study. *Am J Public Health.* 2021;111(10):1851–1854. https://doi.org/10.2105/AJPH.2021.306431

5. Centers for Disease Control and Prevention. CDC WONDER: mortality 1999–2020. Available at: https://wonder.cdc.gov/mcd-icd10.html. Accessed November 3, 2023.
6. Centers for Disease Control and Prevention. CDC WONDER: provisional mortality statistics by multiple cause of death and by single race, for 2018 through present. January 31, 2024. Available at: https://wonder.cdc.gov/wonder/help/mcd-provisional.html. Accessed November 3, 2023.
7. Furr-Holden D, Milam AJ, Wang L, Sadler R. African Americans now outpace Whites in opioid-involved overdose deaths: a comparison of temporal trends from 1999 to 2018. *Addiction.* 2021;116(3): 677–683. https://doi.org/10.1111/add.15233
8. Hoopsick RA, Homish GG, Leonard KE. Differences in opioid overdose mortality rates among middle-aged adults by race/ethnicity and sex, 1999–2018. *Public Health Rep.* 2021;136(2): 192–200. https://doi.org/10.1177/0033354920968806
9. Centers for Disease Control and Prevention. Overdose deaths involving opioids, cocaine, and psychostimulants—United States, 2015–2016. *MMWR Morb Mortal Wkly Rep.* 2018;67(12): 349–358. https://doi.org/10.15585/mmwr.mm6712a1
10. Lopez L III, Hart LH III, Katz MH. Racial and ethnic health disparities related to COVID-19. *JAMA.* 2021;325(8):719–720. https://doi.org/10.1001/jama.2020.26443
11. Gomes T, Ledlie S, Tadrous M, Mamdani M, Paterson JM, Juurlink DN. Trends in opioid toxicity–related deaths in the US before and after the start of the COVID-19 pandemic, 2011–2021. *JAMA Netw Open.* 2023;6(7): e2322303. https://doi.org/10.1001/jamanetworkopen.2023.22303
12. Hammerslag LR, Mack A, Chandler RK, et al. Telemedicine buprenorphine initiation and retention in opioid use disorder treatment for Medicaid enrollees. *JAMA Netw Open.* 2023;6(10): e2336914. https://doi.org/10.1001/jamanetworkopen.2023.36914

Life Expectancy in the United States: A Public Health of Consequence, June 2024

Farzana Kapadia, PhD, MPH

ABOUT THE AUTHOR

Farzana Kapadia is the deputy editor of the American Journal of Public Health *and professor of epidemiology at the School of Global Public Health, New York University, New York, NY.*

See also Woolf, p. 580, Chandra et al., p. 599, Callahan et al., p. 619, and Rempel et al., p. 642.

"The United States is among the wealthiest nations in the world, but it is far from the healthiest."

So begins the summary to the 2013 report *US Health in International Perspective: Shorter Livers, Poorer Health*.[1] It is worth noting, at the outset of this editorial, the title and year of publication of this National Academies of Sciences, Engineering, and Medicine (NASEM) report. This is because more than a decade later, following a period of profound social, economic, political, and public health shocks, on average, Americans live even shorter and unhealthier lives than they did in 2013. Between 2019 and 2022, the main driver of the decline in life expectancy in the United States was COVID-19–related deaths. However, since that time, deaths due to other causes—intentional and unintentional injuries, liver disease, infant and maternal mortality—have persisted, if not increased. Thus, even as COVID-19–related deaths decline, life expectancy in the United States has not rebounded to prepandemic levels. More alarmingly, deaths due to overdose, violence, and other intentional and unintentional injuries persist and, in some cases, continue to increase among younger adults. The result of these outcomes is that people in the United States are living less healthy lives and dying at younger ages than their peers in other Western and high-income countries.

The overall "US health disadvantage," as noted by Woolf and Aron[1] and as long recognized in the public health community, is fueled by the synergistic effects of an underfunded and fragmented public health infrastructure, lack of access to universal health care, and inadequate social, economic, and environmental policies. Underpinning all these drivers are the forces of structural racism and institutional discrimination that fuel inequalities in healthy living and, in turn, racial and ethnic inequities in the risk of dying.

In this issue of the Journal, key articles provide a closer examination of overdose deaths and suicides—two important drivers of lower life expectancy in the United States. Equally important, this editorial highlights an approach that may warrant further adoption across the United States that may prove useful to promoting healthy living across the lifespan for our entire population.

OVERDOSE DEATHS

The US public health crisis of overdose deaths is a uniquely American public health problem. Initially fueled by US-based drug companies pushing opioid pain medication coupled with US physicians' overprescription of opioid pain medication, overdose deaths were further accelerated by the availability of synthetic opioids starting in 2013. Over the past 25 years, the overdose death crisis has had profound ripple effects across US society. A recent study found that more than 40% of US adults personally knew someone who had died from an overdose, and one of eight adults have had their lives disrupted by overdose deaths.[2]

Against this backdrop, there were significant increases in overdose deaths during the pandemic period (https://bit.ly/3IQvzlk). Social, economic, and structural factors such as increasing mental health burdens due to social isolation, job loss, and financial insecurity; lack of access or limited access to substance use treatment programs; and lack of social and family support all contributed to these increases.[3] Recent data from the Centers for Disease Control and Prevention also show that, nationally, race- and ethnicity-based disparities in overdose deaths grew wider during this time period, with Black and African American adults as well as American Indian and Alaskan Native adults experiencing the largest increases in overdose deaths between 2020 and 2021.[4]

We are also aware that from the beginning of the overdose epidemic, overdose deaths have not been evenly distributed across the United States.

To understand whether and how these geographic differences persisted during the pandemic, Chandra et al. (p. 599) present compelling data on the differences in excess overdose mortality during the COVID-19 pandemic by granular geographic area, specifically across US states and counties; they also quantify the burden of excess overdose mortality attributed to specific types of substances, such as synthetic opioids, methamphetamines, alcohol, benzodiazepines, cocaine, and heroin. Their findings provide more evidence for the need to tailor prevention and intervention programs at state and local levels to ensure that the needs of distinct communities are being met. Evidence in support of these recommendations is amplified by Woolf et al. (p. 580), whose report shows that states with stronger economic relief policies saw lower rates of overdose deaths among both men and women.

MONITORING SUICIDE-RELATED DEATHS

In their 2020 editorial, Auerbach and Miller provided a prescient description of how mental health and mental health care delivery would be affected during the COVID-19 pandemic.[5] By highlighting the gaps and inadequacies in mental health care provision, particularly for those already more vulnerable, they called attention to the burdens—social isolation, loneliness, anxiety, and depression—that we now know affected many people directly or indirectly. These burdens and stressors, combined with increased alcohol use and firearm sales, were likely contributors to the increases in suicide, across almost all demographic groups, between 2021 and 2022 (https://bit.ly/3VyJ2Mz).

Recognizing these worrying trends, Ramchand et al. provided a comprehensive set of recommendations to conduct improved monitoring and surveillance of suicide attempts and suicide deaths.[6] Related to this call for enhanced data collection in the context of suicides is a report by Rempel et al. (p. 642) on the need for improved documentation of deaths in the presence of police and law enforcement. By documenting all precustody and in-custody deaths over a 10-year period in Johnson County, Iowa, the authors found that suicide was the cause of over half of trauma-related deaths. Thus, the need for better monitoring of suicide attempts and deaths can provide opportunities for points of intervention and prevention.

SOCIAL CARE FOR LONGER LIVES

We are now well aware that social determinants of health play a major role in influencing individual- and population-level health. Recognizing this early on, many European and high-income countries instituted wide-ranging social and economic reforms to bolster social equity and egalitarianism within their populations. However, similar reforms—such as universal health care—have not been implemented in the United States, and their absence is likely to have contributed to lower life expectancy, higher COVID-19 mortality, and slower rebound in life expectancy to prepandemic levels.

Given the political intransigence to enacting social reforms in the United States, a 2017 NASEM report[7] called for hospitals and health systems to take on the role of anchor institutions by fostering multisectorial partnerships that enhance economic development opportunities for their communities. Such strategies can address social challenges and root causes of poor health and ultimately help shape health equity. Koh et al.[8] previously summarized the challenges and success of some major anchor institutions across the United States that sought to build or leverage community partnerships to increase community benefits and develop assets that positively affect the health and well-being of community members. In 2019, NASEM took one step further and called for health systems to address the social needs of their patients as well as their medical care needs.[9] While recognizing that provision of social care cannot be solved via referral prescriptions alone, there is still value in integrating access to social care within medical care settings. And since integration of these actions often fails because of challenges in system-wide implementation, Callahan et al. (p. 619) report on a case study identifying the practical lessons learned in implementing NASEM's proposed framework for integrating social care and medical care.

In summary, we have the blueprints, operational knowledge, and economic resources to move the social and economic levers that improve health equity. To reverse the US health disadvantage and improve population health, we must embrace bold approaches that can yield the greatest social and economic benefit. AJPH

CORRESPONDENCE

Correspondence should be sent to Farzana Kapadia, PhD, MPH, New York University, School of Global Public Health, 708 Broadway, Room 729, New York, NY 10003 (e-mail: farzana.kapadia@nyu.edu). Reprints can be ordered at http://www.ajph.org by clicking the "Reprints" link.

PUBLICATION INFORMATION

Full Citation: Kapadia F. Life expectancy in the United States: a public health of consequence,

June 2024. *Am J Public Health*. 2024;114(6): 556–558.

Acceptance Date: March 25, 2024

DOI: https://doi.org/10.2105/AJPH.2024.307677

CONFLICTS OF INTEREST

The author has no conflicts of interest to disclose.

REFERENCES

1. National Research Council and Institute of Medicine. *US Health in International Perspective: Shorter Lives, Poorer Health. Panel on Understanding Cross-National Health Differences Among High-Income Countries.* Woolf SH, Aron L, eds. Committee on Population, Division of Behavioral and Social Sciences and Education, and Board on Population Health and Public Health Practice, Institute of Medicine. Washington, DC: National Academies Press; 2013.
2. Athey A, Kilmer B, Cerel J. An overlooked emergency: more than one in eight US adults have had their lives disrupted by drug overdose deaths. *Am J Public Health.* 2024;114(3):276–279. https://doi.org/10.2105/AJPH.2023.307550
3. Tanz LJ, Dinwiddie AT, Snodgrass S, O'Donnell J, Mattson CL, Davis NL. *A Qualitative Assessment of Circumstances Surrounding Drug Overdose Deaths During the Early Stages of the COVID-19 Pandemic.* Atlanta, GA: Centers for Disease Control and Prevention, US Dept of Health and Human Services; 2022. SUDORS Data Brief no. 2.
4. Spencer MR, Miniño AM, Warner M. *Drug Overdose Deaths in the United States, 2001–2021.* Hyattsville, MD: National Center for Health Statistics; 2022. NCHS Data Brief no. 457. https://doi.org/10.15620/cdc:122556
5. Auerbach J, Miller BF. COVID-19 exposes the cracks in our already fragile mental health system. *Am J Public Health.* 2020;110(7):969–970. https://doi.org/10.2105/AJPH.2020.305699
6. Ramchand R, Colpe L, Claassen C, et al. Prioritizing improved data and surveillance for suicide in the United States in response to COVID-19. *Am J Public Health.* 2021;111(S2):S84–S88. https://doi.org/10.2105/AJPH.2021.306258
7. National Academies of Sciences Engineering, Health and Medicine Division, Board on Population Health and Public Health Practice, et al. *Communities in Action: Pathways to Health Equity.* Washington, DC: National Academies Press; 2017.
8. Koh HK, Bantham A, Geller AC, et al. Anchor institutions: best practices to address social needs and social determinants of health. *Am J Public Health.* 2020;110(3):309–316. https://doi.org/10.2105/AJPH.2019.305472
9. National Academies of Sciences Engineering and Medicine (US), Committee on Integrating Social Needs Care Into the Delivery of Health Care to Improve the Nation's Health. *Integrating Social Care Into the Delivery of Health Care: Moving Upstream to Improve the Nation's Health.* Washington, DC: National Academies Press; 2019.

Public Health Legal Protections in an Era of Artificial Intelligence

James G. Hodge Jr, JD, LLM , Jennifer L. Piatt, JD, Erica N. White, JD, and Lawrence O. Gostin, JD

ABOUT THE AUTHORS

James G. Hodge Jr, Jennifer L. Piatt, and Erica N. White are with the Center for Public Health Law and Policy, Sandra Day O'Connor College of Law, Arizona State University, Phoenix. Lawrence O. Gostin is with the O'Neill Institute for Global and National Health Law, Georgetown University Law Center, Washington, DC.

The field of artificial intelligence (AI)—combining computer science and robust data sets to enable problem-solving—offers profound opportunities to improve human health while cutting health care costs. The promises of machine learning to enhance medical diagnoses, speed development and approval of new drugs and vaccines, expedite clinical research, and revolutionize public health surveillance and epidemiological investigations are momentous. Yet, as a new technology with unknown potential, AI is accompanied by significant risks, including medical errors, misinformation, privacy infringements, discrimination, erosion of public trust, and perpetuation of existing health inequities.[1]

The open sourcing of AI portals, beginning with OpenAI's ChatGPT in late 2022, portends new global and national health security threats. Although the predicted catastrophic risks and doomsday scenarios are debatable, without robust protections, AI could endanger public health and safety as law- and policymakers try to catch up to industry capabilities. We assess the public health and security risks of AI applications, examine current law and policy responses, and offer legal guidance to wield AI for population health while mitigating its substantial current and potential harms.

ARTIFICIAL INTELLIGENCE PITFALLS

The publications of an open letter in March 2023 and a brief statement in May signed by industry and tech leaders, academics, and researchers spotlighted catastrophic risks accompanying developing AI technologies.[2] The signatories called for a sustained pause on large AI model development, citing concerns about "an out-of-control race to develop and deploy ever more powerful digital minds."[3] They compared unregulated AI to nuclear war and pandemics.[3] Through documents shared with the US Senate Judiciary Committee on May 16, 2023, OpenAI enunciated possible societal harms of its advanced large language model GPT-4, including disinformation, privacy infringements, cybersecurity risks, "harmful content," and the "proliferation of conventional and unconventional weapons."[3] Additional forewarnings included the possibility for (1) manipulation of AI technologies for subversive ends, (2) displacement of humans via technological efficiencies (which Google purportedly endorsed in November 2023, asking governments to develop "global AI corps"), (3) prioritization of corporate profits over public safety, and (4) superintelligent AI applications exceeding human control.[4]

These risks may jeopardize the public's health in manifold ways. Transgressors are already using AI for propaganda generation, threatening democratic institutions and elections. Online misinformation substantially influenced US national elections in 2016 and 2020.[5] AI tools are projected to affect election integrity further in 2024, amplifying mis- and disinformation.[6] AI tendencies to "hallucinate" (i.e., fabricate inaccurate responses to queries) or reflect specific political viewpoints are problematic absent widespread public knowledge about the technology's limitations. Voters' tarnished trust in election results may be compounded by AI, potentially leading to governmental instability, violence, and public health upheaval.

AI applications may provide factually inaccurate or discriminatory information to specific users. In a widely publicized example emerging in June 2023, the National Eating Disorders Association replaced a human-staffed helpline with an AI chatbot. The chatbot began providing requesters with inappropriate dieting advice, which might have contributed to eating disorders.[7] Generative AI responds to questions based on data it is trained on, some of which may have been acquired unethically (e.g., without adequate informed consent). Prejudiced or discriminatory responses from chatbots reflect biases and inequities. Chatbots have issued statements categorizing "Black men as criminals 10% more than White men" and "tend[ing] to classify women as homemakers over White men."[8(p6)]

Enabling technologies containing biases to provide health-based advice or public health data without counter-protections endangers individuals and the community. The Food and Drug Administration (FDA) commissioner Robert Califf has intimated repeatedly how health misinformation contributes to lower US life expectancies.[9] Social media is already rife with misinformation about disease spread, vaccines, and medical treatment as experienced during the COVID-19 pandemic. Imagine the global repercussions of human responses to real-time misinformation generated through AI-infused data centers during a future pandemic or natural disaster.

Additionally, significant AI risks arise from the potential development and proliferation of lethal autonomous weapons systems through domestic and foreign militaries. Ongoing global conflicts are testing grounds for semiautonomous drones and "counter-drone weapons endowed with AI."[10] Fully autonomous AI-laden drones may soon be used to "identify, select, and attack targets without help from humans."[11] Although the US Department of Defense has indicated it will not withdraw human control over AI military technologies, other nations and private entities may not follow suit.[11] Significant concerns over unpredictable drone strikes or detonations would heighten exponentially if malicious private actors steal and use military AI technologies.

NAVIGATING RISKS

Public and private sources largely concur that existing laws and policies in the United States and abroad insufficiently protect against AI risks to public health and safety. Where AI executives and government leaders diverge is on how, precisely, to regulate an industry that defies boundaries and is constantly advancing. Global assessments, such as the World Health Organization's 2021 report on AI in health care, are already outdated and lack enforcement mechanisms.[12] The European Union's (EU's) Artificial Intelligence Act, proposed in 2021 and expected to be finalized in 2024, may be the first comprehensive governance mechanism for regulating AI.[13] Framing product regulation rather than human rights, the act would generally prohibit "unacceptable risk" of vaguely defined AI technologies "considered to be a clear threat to people's safety, livelihoods and rights."[13] Some closely regulated, high-risk AI uses concern public health, such as reliance on AI for product safety and public service access.[13] What else might be captured under the act's coverage, however, is indeterminate.

Acting with increasing urgency to expedite the regulation of AI technologies, US Congress members seek to balance societal protections with technological innovations pushed by the massive US tech industry. Several bills introduced in 2023 would establish affirmative duties for AI companies to assess their products, require transparency when AI is used, allow more robust regulations based on expanded jurisdiction and oversight, and prohibit the distribution of certain AI-generated images.[14] Meaningful federal legislation, however, is many months away from bipartisan passage and enactment and likely years from implementation.

Even as tech giants publicly call for strong governmental oversight, they oppose large-scale legal reforms of their expansive models. Sam Altman, the embattled chief executive of OpenAI who equates AI access with human empowerment, has suggested that regulations apply only to future AI uses, not current ones. In May 2023, he asserted that compliance with the EU's pending regulations would cause the company to cease operations overseas.[15] In late July, multiple technology companies formed the Frontier Model Forum to provide industry-led guidance on mitigating AI safety threats and immoral uses. Still, they actively resist governmental alliances, including an October agreement among G7 nations and the November Bletchley Declaration among the United Kingdom, the United States, China, and 24 other countries, which promises to closely monitor the industry.

On October 30, 2023, President Joe Biden signed a new executive order in follow-up to his administration's Blueprint for an AI Bill of Rights. Regulatory objectives outlined in the executive order include (1) processes to mitigate AI adoption risks among more than 30 federal entities, (2) equity and civil rights considerations concerning criminal justice and government programs administration, (3) consumer protections and worker support, and (4) US global regulatory leadership and innovation.[16] The executive order legitimizes Federal Trade Commission jurisdiction over AI based on existing statutory authorities, including antitrust and anticompetitiveness.[17] On November 1, 2023, Vice President Kamala Harris announced the US AI Safety Institute, which operationalized the National Institute of Standards and Technology AI Risk Management Framework to enforce previous voluntary guidelines and best practices.[17]

The Department of Health and Human Services and the FDA have committed to patients' safety and health while supporting AI innovations.[18]

Accommodating these potentially divergent interests is complicated. Existing FDA guidance on medical technologies, for example, may apply to AI uses but does not sufficiently account for novel risks in substituting technological findings for clinicians' assessments. Although AI medical applications may already be more accurate than clinicians in specific cases (e.g., colon cancer screenings), overreliance on AI-generated diagnoses or treatments can harm the public's health, particularly through identified biases, including using debunked race-based equations or assessments.[19]

Lacking comprehensive federal guidance, state legislatures have attempted to regulate AI technologies through patchwork approaches echoing, in part, the EU model. Between January 1 and September 27, 2023, 27 states and Washington, DC, introduced AI-related legislation.[20] Twenty bills in 15 states have passed centered on overall transparency and accountability, public disclosure of AI uses, and data use limits based largely on consumer privacy protections.[20] Some state legislatures have considered select public health repercussions of AI. Bills in California, for example, seek to address mental health risks and prohibit health insurance discrimination associated with AI uses.[20] Alabama, Hawaii, New Jersey, and Vermont have established novel agencies or departments to assess AI and craft future policies and procedures.[20] State-by-state approaches could undermine uniform national regulatory responses called for by the President and Congress.

LEGAL PROTECTIONS

Avoiding harm to public health and safety from AI is vital. Existing legal measures designed to protect privacy, avoid discrimination, ensure equitable distributions of health resources, and identify or mitigate catastrophic threats may not adequately regulate potentially harmful AI applications. Enhanced legal and policy approaches are warranted.

Tens of millions of US residents using AI chatbots in the past year alone are aware of some of the chatbots' utilities but not necessarily their limitations and biases. Existing standards to raise consumer awareness of technological functions tend to seek informed consent and releases of liability through electronic agreements executed before use. Similar requirements applied to AI chatbots are dubious. Individuals already beleaguered with constant prompts to click their assent to long, fine-print requirements for online use or access are unlikely to scrutinize disclaimers before seeking answers from generative AI. Such mandates could be retailored to require active learning tutorials on the benefits and risks of AI. Even though consumers likely cannot negotiate their own terms of use, options to set or enable filters (e.g., identifying hallucinated results and using clear watermarks that identify AI-generated images, as required in President Biden's executive order) can help them digest the quality and accuracy of generated information. What AI users cannot currently choose, however, is how such technologies may be used against them based, in part, on their own data mined online. It is essential to have strong adherence to existing civil protections under an array of federal and state laws prohibiting privacy infringements and unwarranted discrimination tied to AI data collections and uses.

When specific commercial products or services propagate false, harmful, or dangerous information, regulators can limit harm. In May 2023, the Federal Trade Commission asserted its authority to regulate large language model neural AI networks to the extent they deceive consumers and affect fair competition. Additional federal and state consumer safety agencies may intervene as well to monitor, regulate, recall, and require public notices of injurious facets of AI technologies. In fall 2023, President Biden and Senator Chuck Schumer advocated imposing "duty of care" requirements on the industry to essentially police itself under threat of sanctions. The tsunami of AI misinformation demonstrates the need for legal requirements for technology companies to closely assess their products, ensure active collaboration with public health authorities, and publicize notices of harmful practices and data sharing injurious to communal health.

Sensational fears that AI applications could contribute to or cause catastrophic public health events, including human subjugation, disruption of essential systems (e.g., water supply[21]) or resources, and augmentation of existing threats, justify advanced global and national security protections.[22] US officials must wield powers responsibly and ethically, balancing potential harms with infringements of free speech and other constitutional rights. Along the AI threat spectrum is the potential for generated misinformation to influence specific users or entire subpopulations to undertake risky behaviors (e.g., inappropriate dieting techniques) or avoid safe ones (e.g., administration of efficacious vaccines). Advanced measures to limit AI chatbot outputs may be warranted, especially where the health of minors or other vulnerable populations is endangered.

A new type of public health emergency centered on human or electronic surveillance of critical impacts of widespread misinformation may trigger real-time requirements for AI companies to scrub or recall such data from their programs. Social media and tech companies have previously worked internally to clean up their sites (e.g., removing antivaccination falsehoods or highly discriminatory content) but may still resist emergency governmental mandates, asserting First Amendment commercial speech protections. The US Supreme Court has clarified, however, that such protections do not extend to propagating false or misleading information that harms the public's health.[23] The US government can require rapid industry corrections of AI platforms amid emergency declarations. Pursuant to President Biden's executive order, the Defense Production Act may be evoked to regulate AI models implicating national security that affects the public's health.

Corporations introducing products or services to the United States or global markets that directly harm individuals or populations are generally liable for damages. Why should AI companies be treated any differently? Multiple class action lawsuits against the industry have already been filed claiming chatbots improperly mined copyrighted online data.[24] Employers including Apple Inc. have restricted employee uses of generative AI at work to avoid proprietary information uploads. Additional cases alleging defamation, medical malpractice, and other direct harms to consumers have surfaced as well.

Tech giants, however, may have a defense against generalized claims that AI applications harm populations. Under existing federal statutory law, companies enjoy a level of immunity from allegations that data posted or accessed on their sites have been used for invidious ends. On May 18, 2023, the Supreme Court refused to extend liability to Twitter (or X) against claims that its media contributed to terroristic acts. In the absence of "knowing" and "substantial" action, the company was found not liable for "aiding and abetting" a terrorist organization by merely allowing known, affiliated users on its platform.[25]

AI providers may similarly deny responsibility for harmful uses or outcomes. Such specious reasoning has been perpetuated in other public health legal arenas (e.g., "guns don't kill people"; "opioids are not dangerous unless consumers misuse them"). This type of reasoning may not hold up concerning AI chatbots that providers already acknowledge produce biased, hallucinated, incorrect, and even dangerous information. In light of projected harms stemming from a massive quantity of false data generated through AI applications, the Supreme Court may reconsider the scope of existing federal liability protections. Coextensively, it is also reviewing First Amendment limits of government-led interventions to require social media companies to remove, or keep in place, misinformation or specific viewpoints on their sites. Forthcoming decisions in these opposing cases may clarify the reach of governmental regulation and liability for false or misleading information propagated through AI chatbots.

CONCLUSIONS

The irreversible rise of AI ushers in an era of an explosive number of new applications presenting abundant benefits coupled with preventable harms to the public's health. Human health and safety are not trade-offs in the interests of economics or profits. As industry leaders and others have championed, ensuring the health and security of populations domestically and abroad is essential for avoiding potentially catastrophic outcomes. AJPH

CORRESPONDENCE

Correspondence should be sent to James G. Hodge Jr, JD, LLM, Sandra Day O'Connor College of Law, Arizona State University, 111 E. Taylor St, MC 9520, Phoenix, AZ 85004 (e-mail: james.hodge.1@asu.edu). Reprints can be ordered at http://www.ajph.org by clicking the "Reprints" link.

PUBLICATION INFORMATION

Full Citation: Hodge JG Jr, Piatt JL, White EN, Gostin LO. Public health legal protections in an era of artificial intelligence. *Am J Public Health.* 2024;114(6):559–563.

Acceptance Date: January 26, 2024.

DOI: https://doi.org/10.2105/AJPH.2024.307619

CONTRIBUTORS

J. G. Hodge Jr supervised and all authors contributed to the conceptualization, research, drafting, and editing of the article.

ACKNOWLEDGMENTS

The views expressed in this article are those of the authors and not necessarily those of their institutions.

CONFLICTS OF INTEREST

The authors have no financial, personal, academic, or other conflicts of interest in the subject matter discussed in this article.

REFERENCES

1. Lekadir K, Quaglio G, Tselioudis Garmendia A, Gallin C. *Artificial Intelligence in Healthcare: Applications, Risks, and Ethical and Societal Impacts.* Luxembourg, Luxembourg: European Parliament; 2022. https://doi.org/10.2861/568473
2. Roose K. AI poses "risk of extinction," industry leaders warn. *New York Times.* May 30, 2023. Available at: https://www.nytimes.com/2023/05/30/technology/ai-threat-warning.html. Accessed November 27, 2023.
3. US Senate Committee on the Judiciary. Oversight of A.I.: rules for artificial intelligences. March 23, 2023. Available at: https://www.judiciary.senate.gov/committee-activity/hearings/oversight-of-ai-rules-for-artificial-intelligence. Accessed November 27, 2023.
4. Center for AI Safety. Risks from AI: an overview of catastrophic AI risks. Available at: https://www.safe.ai/ai-risk. Accessed November 27, 2023.
5. Moore RC, Dahlke R, Hancock JT. Exposure to untrustworthy websites in the 2020 US election. *Nat Hum Behav.* 2023;7(7):1096–1105. https://doi.org/10.1038/s41562-023-01564-2
6. Ulmer A, Tong A. Deepfaking it: America's 2024 election collides with AI boom. May 30, 2023. Available at: https://www.reuters.com/world/us/

deepfaking-it-americas-2024-election-collides-with-ai-boom-2023-05-30. Accessed November 27, 2023.

7. McCarthy L. A wellness chatbot is offline after its "harmful" focus on weight loss. *New York Times*. June 9, 2023. Available at: https://www.nytimes.com/2023/06/08/us/ai-chatbot-tessa-eating-disorders-association.html. Accessed November 27, 2023.
8. Getahun H. ChatGPT could be used for good, but like many other AI models, it's rife with racist and discriminatory bias. *Insider*. January 16, 2023. Available at: https://www.insider.com/chatgpt-is-like-many-other-ai-models-rife-with-bias-2023-1. Accessed March 30, 2024.
9. Tirrell M. Health misinformation is lowering US life expectancy, FDA commissioner Robert Califf says. April 12, 2023. Available at: https://www.cnbc.com/2023/04/11/us-life-expectancy-hurt-by-misinformation-fda-commissioner-robert-califf.html. Accessed November 27, 2023.
10. Bajak F, Arhirova H. Drone advances amid war in Ukraine could bring fighting robots to front lines. *PBS Newshour*. January 3, 2023. Available at: https://www.pbs.org/newshour/world/drone-advances-amid-war-in-ukraine-could-bring-fighting-robots-to-front-lines. Accessed November 27, 2023.
11. Hudson J, Khudov K. The war in Ukraine is spurring a revolution in drone warfare using AI. *Washington Post*. July 26, 2023. Available at: https://www.washingtonpost.com/world/2023/07/26/drones-ai-ukraine-war-innovation. Accessed November 27, 2023.
12. World Health Organization. WHO calls for safe and ethical AI for health. May 16, 2023. Available at: https://www.who.int/news/item/16-05-2023-who-calls-for-safe-and-ethical-ai-for-health. Accessed November 27, 2023.
13. Madiega T. Briefing: EU legislation in progress: artificial intelligence act. June 2023. Available at: https://www.europarl.europa.eu/RegData/etudes/BRIE/2021/698792/EPRS_BRI(2021)698792_EN.pdf. Accessed November 27, 2023.
14. Brennan Center for Justice. Artificial intelligence legislation tracker. August 7, 2023. Available at: https://www.brennancenter.org/our-work/research-reports/artificial-intelligence-legislation-tracker. Accessed November 27, 2023.
15. Waters R, Murgia M, Espinoza J. OpenAI warns over split with Europe as regulation advances. *Financial Times*. May 25, 2023. Available at: https://www.ft.com/content/5814b408-8111-49a9-8885-8a8434022352. Accessed November 27, 2023.
16. Executive Order 14100 of October 30, 2023. Safe, secure, and trustworthy development and use of artificial intelligence. *Fed Regist*. 2023;88(210):75191–75226. Available at: https://www.federalregister.gov/documents/2023/11/01/2023-24283/safe-secure-and-trustworthy-development-and-use-of-artificial-intelligence. Accessed November 27, 2023.
17. White House. Fact sheet: Vice President Harris announces new US initiatives to advance the safe and responsible use of artificial intelligence. November 1, 2023. Available at: https://www.whitehouse.gov/briefing-room/statements-releases/2023/11/01/fact-sheet-vice-president-harris-announces-new-u-s-initiatives-to-advance-the-safe-and-responsible-use-of-artificial-intelligence. Accessed November 27, 2023.
18. Chung J. How will health care regulators address artificial intelligence? *Regulatory Review*. October 18, 2021. Available at: https://www.theregreview.org/2021/10/18/chung-how-will-health-care-regulators-address-artificial-intelligence. Accessed November 27, 2023.
19. Goldman M. Study: some AI chatbots provide racist health info. *Axios*. October 23, 2023. Available at: https://www.axios.com/2023/10/23/ai-chatbot-racism-medicine. Accessed November 27, 2023.
20. National Conference of State Legislatures. Summary: artificial intelligence 2023 legislation. July 20, 2023. Available at: https://www.ncsl.org/technology-and-communication/artificial-intelligence-2023-legislation. Accessed November 27, 2023.
21. Richards CE, Tzachor A, Avin S, Fenner R. Rewards, risks and responsible deployment of artificial intelligence in water systems. *Nature Water*. 2023;1:422–432. https://doi.org/10.1038/s44221-023-00069-6
22. Federspiel F, Mitchell R, Asokan A, Umana C, McCoy D. Threats by artificial intelligence to human health and human existence. *BMJ Glob Health*. 2023;8(5):e010435. https://doi.org/10.1136/bmjgh-2022-010435
23. *Central Hudson Gas & Electric Corp. v Public Service Commission*, 447 US 557 (1980).
24. De Vynck G. ChatGPT maker OpenAI faces a lawsuit over how it used people's data. *Washington Post*. June 28, 2023. Available at: https://www.washingtonpost.com/technology/2023/06/28/openai-chatgpt-lawsuit-class-action. Accessed November 27, 2023.
25. *Twitter, Inc., et al. v Mehier Taamneh, et al.*, 598 US 471 (2023).

On the Appearance and Disappearance of Difficult Medical Histories: What Does It Take to Sustain Public Memory?

Susan M. Reverby, PhD, and Amy Moran-Thomas, PhD

ABOUT THE AUTHORS

Susan M. Reverby is with Women's and Gender Studies, Wellesley College, Wellesley, MA. Amy Moran-Thomas is with the Department of Anthropology, Massachusetts Institute of Technology, Cambridge.

AJPH June 2024, Vol. 114, No. 6

More than a decade has passed since the *AJPH* essay "First, Do No Harm"[1] joined other robust media coverage and scholarship on the unsettling findings of a US-sponsored inoculation study of sexually transmitted infections in Guatemala, conducted between 1946 and 1948 without informed consent or extensive treatment (Box 1). The majority of the subjects targeted in these unethical experiments were Indigenous people. One of us (S. M. R.) uncovered these disturbing records in the course of archival research (Figure 1). The article describing this, "'Normal Exposure' and Inoculation Syphilis: A PHS 'Tuskegee' Doctor in Guatemala," given to the Centers for Disease Control and Prevention (CDC) before publication in 2010, led to the Obama administration's apology to Guatemala, and the subsequent federal bioethics reports.[2–4] Amid an all-too-brief surge of public attention to the facts of the case, Rodriguez and García's essay in *AJPH* contributed an important reflection from a bioethical and legal perspective.[1] They joined the many public scholars working to envision what remedies might look like in response to such an obviously egregious historical injustice.

With the passage of time, it is striking that none of these suggested remediations have happened—most have not even been publicly attempted. Rodriguez and García carefully laid out the logistics of how those who were harmed in the Guatemala experiments might be compensated, building on the US Public Health Service's Study of Untreated Syphilis in Tuskegee as a model (although because of the international nature of the Guatemala case, this would require waiving sovereign immunity). But the US government never created Rodriguez and García's recommended compensation program to

> more concretely and permanently acknowledge the wrongful nature of the conduct in question, in keeping with the expressive function of both US and international law.[5]

Their 2013 commentary also noted that

> the Centers for Disease Control and Prevention was tasked with developing a case study on the unethical research conducted in Guatemala. The study will include learning objectives focused on scientific and ethical issues in designing a field investigation.[1(p2123)]

Today, we have not been able to locate any such public-facing document from the CDC. Likewise, it was also hoped that the Collaborative Institutional Training Initiative (CITI) required as part of institutional review board certification would add some content about the Guatemala events, as part of educating future researchers. One of us (S. M. R.) was in touch with CITI about this back in 2014. But these changes to CITI modules seem to have not materialized.

Nor have other sectors of the federal government responded to other concerns the experiments in Guatemala raised. For example, legal scholars have called for the US government to conduct a public stocktaking of what happened to the blood and tissue samples extracted from people in the course of these experiments, to clarify what ultimately became of these biospecimens, and to return any samples of blood or tissue that might still be in the possession of federal institutions such as the National Institutes of Health (NIH).[6] This does not seem to have been carried out. The Presidential Commission for

BOX 1— The US Public Health Service Sexually Transmitted Disease (STD) Experiments in Guatemala, 1946–1948

Brief Facts

Between 1946 and 1948, researchers from the US Public Health Service in conjunction with the Guatemalan Ministry of Health intentionally infected at least 1308 people in Guatemala with syphilis, gonorrhea, and chancroid. They conducted serology tests on about 3820 others. Results of the studies were kept secret and never published.

Most of the people experimented on were Indigenous people. Doctors estimated that 85% of the population of Guatemala City at the time was Maya. They also traveled to places they imagined as being entirely Maya or otherwise racialized to study their theories of "racial immunity."

The experiments were to see in part if the newly discovered penicillin could serve as a prophylaxis, not just a cure, for early venereal diseases, and to refine formulas and dosage. Done without consent, the studies began by hiring sex workers (many infected by the study doctors) to have intercourse with prisoners in the Guatemala City federal prison. Other experiments included inoculations into genitalia, spines, and arms, as well as blood tests, conducted without consent from "subjects" in an orphanage, a mental asylum, an army barracks, and with additional sex workers.

A previous study in the United States was unable to consistently produce gonorrhea infections in prisoners at a federal Terre Haute, Indiana, prison through inoculations. Because bringing sex workers into the prison in Guatemala was legal, this new study began there since it allowed for what the researchers called "normal exposure." It expanded to the other sites in Guatemala.

Some study "subjects" in Guatemala were egregiously physically violated, although it is unclear exactly how many deaths were directly caused by the experiments, and how many people really became infected, or were treated.

Despite the dictum "to do no harm," and the Nuremberg code of research ethics being articulated against Nazi human experimenters at the same time (1947), researchers from the United States claimed that their secretive experiments were justified as part of the "war on syphilis" and other STDs.

The principal investigator in Guatemala later worked on the untreated syphilis studies in Tuskegee, Alabama (where African American men who had late-stage syphilis were denied treatment and followed for four decades). In both these studies, the researchers' actions were immoral, did not use consented procedures, and mostly did not include treatment for study subjects, although researchers wrongly claimed they had provided treatment.

While more than a dozen studies of the work in Tuskegee were published, the experiments in Guatemala were kept secret. Knowledge of the study in Tuskegee has circulated for more than half a century, in contrast to the Guatemala case. Despite media coverage in 2010, commission reports from the US and Guatemalan governments, and various court cases, many US public and health professionals are still largely unaware of these experiments in Guatemala and the lack of reparations, compensation, and access to justice through the courts for those who were injured.

What Was Proposed and Has Been Left Undone

- A US government compensation and reparation program that compensates surviving participants for the injuries sustained and those secondarily infected for direct harms (e.g., disease transmission) as well as indirect harms (e.g., emotional distress, loss of a family member at a younger age), and that acknowledges "the wrongful nature of the conduct in question." The program could follow the model and payment structure used to compensate study subjects and families affected by the syphilis experiment in Tuskegee. Such a compensation program could be created by the US federal government and administered by its agencies. Just recently, the CDC Foundation has offered $5 million for the education of the descendants of the men in the Tuskegee study.
- Appropriate medical treatment and historical acknowledgement for those harmed across generations, with support from the US institutions and universities that were involved.
- A proposed CDC case study carried out to document an agency perspective "on the unethical research conducted in Guatemala, with learning objectives focused on scientific and ethical issues in designing a field investigation."
- Integration of the Guatemala Study into researcher training, such as the CITI course required by IRBs, including acknowledgement that Indigenous people were disproportionately harmed.
- A call for the NIH to account for the study's biospecimens, or to acknowledge if they were misplaced or destroyed. If blood or tissue are located, they should be returned to communities.
- A more concerted effort to inform the public, acknowledging both the difficulty of such historical facts in perpetuating distrust and the necessity of this step for trust in the future.

Note. CDC = Centers for Disease Control and Prevention; CITI = Collaborative Institutional Training Initiative; IRB = institutional review board; NIH = National Institutes of Health.
Source. Rodriguez and García,[1] and Reverby.[2]

the Study of Bioethical Issues that summarized the facts of the case in 2011 was meant, at the time, to be a stepping stone toward more concrete future remedies ahead. Instead, it currently stands as a marker of a deeply unfinished response.[4] No subsequent presidential administrations have restarted a bioethics commission to more fully address next steps, including fundamental questions about what those harmed might be owed.[5]

Unsurprisingly, given all this, the search for justice has ended up in the courts. After the first case in the US federal government was dismissed in 2011 for reasons of sovereign immunity, the US government never arranged another form of settlement for affected families in Guatemala. (It did provide money to the Guatemalan government for sexually transmitted infection care in general, as Rodriguez and García noted in their analysis of why this step alone is insufficient.[1]) A subsequent case (*Estate of Arturo Giron Alvarez et al. v The Johns Hopkins University et al.*) was brought against Johns Hopkins, the Rockefeller Foundation, and the pharmaceutical company Bristol Myers

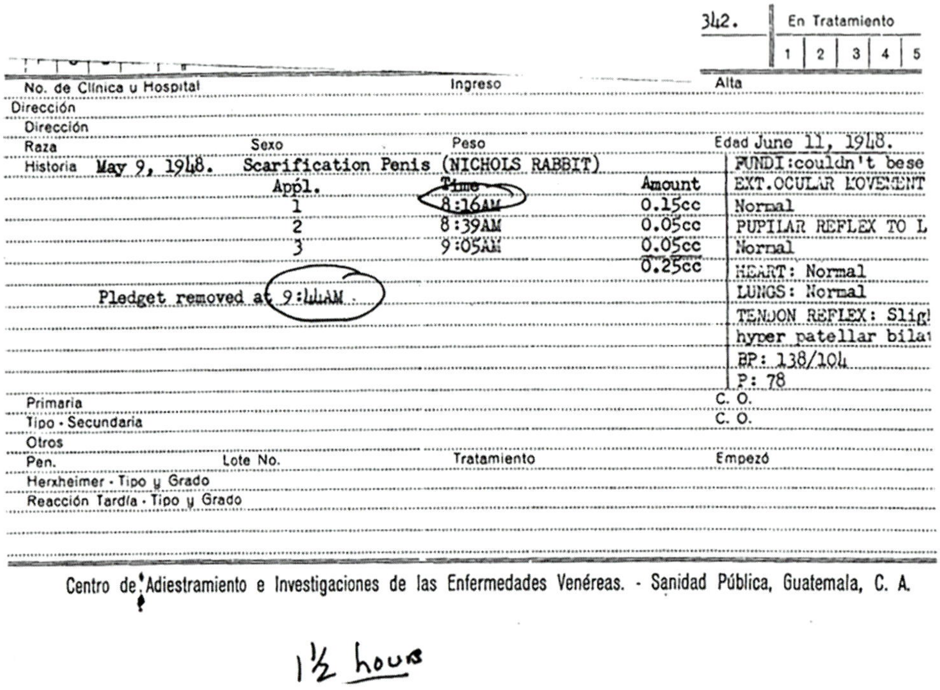
342. En Tratamiento 1 2 3 4 5

No. de Clínica u Hospital Ingreso Alta
Dirección
Dirección
Raza Sexo Peso Edad June 11, 1948.
Historia May 9, 1948. Scarification Penis (NICHOLS RABBIT)
Appl. Time Amount
1 8:16AM 0.15cc
2 8:39AM 0.05cc
3 9:05AM 0.05cc
0.25cc
Pledget removed at 9:44AM.

FUNDI: couldn't bese
EXT. OCULAR MOVEMENT
Normal
PUPILAR REFLEX TO L
Normal
HEART: Normal
LUNGS: Normal
TENDON REFLEX: Sligl
hyper patellar bila
BP: 138/104
P: 78

Primaria C. O.
Tipo - Secundaria C. O.
Otros
Pen. Lote No. Tratamiento Empezó
Herxheimer - Tipo y Grado
Reacción Tardía - Tipo y Grado

Centro de Adiestramiento e Investigaciones de las Enfermedades Venéreas. - Sanidad Pública, Guatemala, C. A.

1½ hours

FIGURE 1— Sample Medical Record From the US Public Health Service Sexually Transmitted Disease (STD) Experiments in Guatemala, 1946–1948

Note. The handwritten note on amount of time is by author Susan M. Reverby.
Source. John C. Cutler Papers, University of Pittsburgh Archives, now in the National Archives South East Regional Archives, Morrow, GA, RG 442; online at https://www.archives.gov/research/health/cdc-cutler-records.

Squibb in 2015, as families in Guatemala searched for restitution from a much less clear-cut constellation of institutional actors involved at the time. One of us (S. M. R.) testified as a historian in the case, wanting to bring more public attention to Guatemalan families' efforts to seek justice, even while acknowledging there are no easy answers to the many difficult questions raised in the absence of governmental accountability. Media and scholarly attention to the stakes of the case has been relatively muted; at the time of writing, the *Alvarez* case is on appeal to the 4th Circuit, argued in December 2023 with no decision to date. When one of us (A. M.-T.), who attended the 2016 opening hearings, taught about the case in a bioethics unit last year, not a single student in the class had heard about the experiments in Guatemala.

It is worth considering why the study in Tuskegee has continued to have so much cultural resonance in the United States, while the Guatemala story has faded. It has been more than 50 years since the study in Tuskegee ended, a longer time for it to be enshrined in public memory, scholarship, music, and fiction.[7–9] It became a key part of the US bioethics cannon of cautionary cases warning researchers about "racism in research,"[10] after Congressional hearings, a federal report, and a lawsuit. Yet making that study into an exemplary case took decades and then organizing by historians, health advocates, and Black political figures before the federal apology finally happened in 1997, 25 years after the study ended.[11]

The case was often called to memory in Black communities and by journalists during the AIDS epidemic and again during the recent COVID-19 pandemic, as shorthand for the layered reasons many non-White populations have to distrust medical authorities.[12,13] And today, the study's memory is also carried forward in powerfully agentive ways by the descendants of the study's unwitting participants.[14] In short, it was not the facts of the case alone, but also the ways that people and institutions created relationships and practices around them over time that shaped its place in memory.

These facts remind us that collective relationships and persistence both matter—and can be all too necessary—for how history becomes known. This is true on the governmental level—but also, of course, for the collective pressures and public advocacy that state agencies tend to respond to. Indeed, connections growing out of responses to the study in Tuskegee were foundational in bringing the Guatemala case to light in the first place, offering lessons for work still ahead. The research by one of us (S. M. R.) for her book on the study in Tuskegee led to her finding the Guatemala materials, which otherwise might have gone unattended to until now. She already had connections to former CDC Director David Sencer, whom she'd been interviewing for her research about his role at the CDC during the time of the study in Tuskegee, which led to the federal involvement in the response to her work on the Guatemala experiments. The CDC, the NIH, the US Domestic Policy Council at the White House, the State Department's consideration of the consequences of the public exposure of these experiments, and the CDC's leadership's connection to health policy guru Zeke Emanuel in the Obama administration, all then led to the apology.[15] The government response might have unfolded very differently without this contingent context.

And, of course, the ongoing legacies of these historical experiments are hardly forgotten in Guatemala—certainly not by the families living with its sequelae. Certain chronic conditions given to people in Guatemala by US researchers can be passed (especially during pregnancy) between generations.[16] This means there are still children being born with these pathogens in their bodies today—a disturbing manifestation of much larger questions about how historical harms can live on, and the need to address them across generations. Today there is increasing attention to the fact that a majority of those targeted were Indigenous people, at a time when rising consciousness about the interlocking faces of scientific racism is generating growing solidarities around the world, which may coalesce still other collective responses ahead.[17–19]

Like the study in Tuskegee, the chapter of research misconduct from Guatemala is also a reminder that the struggle for recognition of such ethical violations is never just a one-time revelation of new data. It takes media coverage and public activation—including scholarly attention to lived realities—to give information meaning and to galvanize institutional responses.[20] This memory work for the experiments in Guatemala is still ongoing and growing. Together with scholars across Guatemala and the United States, we hope to continue participating in its futures.

This 10-year retrospective invites us all to ask what our own roles may be in transforming these events into an example that might be better grieved, publicly responded to, and acknowledged by our institutions in the present. Looking back on Rodriguez and García's essay—full of persuasive, unheeded recommendations—is a sobering reminder of all the work still ahead. We must collectively try to attend to how such histories live in the present and continue to shape our shared future. AJPH

CORRESPONDENCE

Correspondence should be sent to Susan M. Reverby, Women's and Gender Studies Department, Wellesley College, 106 Central St, Wellesley, MA 02481 (e-mail: sreverby@wellesley.edu). Reprints can be ordered at http://www.ajph.org by clicking the "Reprints" link.

PUBLICATION INFORMATION

Full Citation: Reverby SM, Moran-Thomas A. On the appearance and disappearance of difficult medical histories: what does it take to sustain public memory? *Am J Public Health*. 2024;114(6): 564–568.

Acceptance Date: February 23, 2024

DOI: https://doi.org/10.2105/AJPH.2024.307643

CONTRIBUTORS

Both authors conceptualized, wrote, and edited the contribution together.

ACKNOWLEDGMENTS

These reflections grew in part from an earlier presentation at the Harvard Weatherhead Friday Morning Seminar in Culture, Psychiatry and Global Mental Health.

We are grateful to the seminar organizers and participants for a lively conversation that fed this article, with special thanks to Martín Rangel for offering updates from Guatemala and to MIT Anthropology for their support.

CONFLICTS OF INTEREST

The authors report no conflicts of interest.

REFERENCES

1. Rodriguez MA, García R. First, do no harm: the US sexually transmitted disease experiments in Guatemala. *Am J Public Health*. 2013;103(12): 2122–2126. https://doi.org/10.2105/AJPH.2013.301520
2. Reverby SM. "Normal exposure" and inoculation syphilis: a PHS "Tuskegee" doctor in Guatemala, 1946–1948. *J Policy Hist*. 2011;23(1):6–28. https://doi.org/10.1017/S0898030610000291
3. McNeil DG. US apologizes for syphilis tests in Guatemala. *New York Times*. October 1, 2010:1.
4. Presidential Commission for the Study of Bioethical Issues. "Ethically impossible" STD research in Guatemala from 1946 to 1948. 2011. Available at: https://bioethicsarchive.georgetown.edu/pcsbi/node/654.html. Accessed March 12, 2024.
5. Gavin M. NAS and NAM presidents, other experts urge Biden administration to reinstate Presidential Bioethics Commission. National Academies, March 2, 2022, Available at: https://www.nationalacademies.org/news/2022/03/nas-and-nam-presidents-other-experts-urge-biden-administration-to-reinstate-presidential-bioethics-commission. Accessed March 12, 2024.
6. Spector-Bagdady K, Lombardo P. From in vivo to in vitro: how the Guatemala STD experiments transformed bodies into biospecimens. *Milbank Q*. 2018;96(2):244–271. https://doi.org/10.1111/1468-0009.12318
7. Frazier C. It's more than just news: print media, the Tuskegee Syphilis Study and collective memory among African Americans. *Sociology Lens*. 2020;33(3):280–296.
8. Jones JH. *Bad Blood*. New York, NY: Free Press, 1981.
9. Reverby SM. *Examining Tuskegee: The Infamous Syphilis Study and Its Legacy*. Chapel Hill, NC: University of North Carolina Press; 2009.
10. Brandt AM. Racism and research: the case of the Tuskegee Syphilis study. *Hastings Cent Rep*. 1978;8(6):21–29. https://doi.org/10.2307/3561468
11. Harter L, Stephans R, Japp P. President Clinton's apology for the Tuskegee Syphilis Experiment. *Howard J Commun*. 2000;11(1):19–34. https://doi.org/10.1080/106461700246698

12. Thomas SB, Quinn SC. The Tuskegee Syphilis Study, 1932 to 1972: implications for HIV education and AIDS risk education programs in the black community. *Am J Public Health*. 1991;81(11):1498–1505. https://doi.org/10.2105/AJPH.81.11.1498

13. Hammonds EM, Reverby SM. Taking a medical history: COVID, "mistrust," and racism. The Mudsill 1. April 15, 2021. Available at: https://themudsill.substack.com/p/the-mudsill-vol-1-no-7. Accessed March 12, 2024.

14. Voices of our Fathers Legacy Foundation. 2024. Available at: https://www.voicesforfathers.org. Accessed March 12, 2024.

15. Reverby SM. Ethical failures and history lessons: the US Public Health Service research studies in Tuskegee and Guatemala. *Public Health Rev*. 2012;34(1):1–18. https://doi.org/10.1007/BF03391665

16. Crafts L. Making medical subjects: regeneration, experimentation, and women in the Guatemalan spring. *Hisp Am Hist Rev*. 2022;102(2):251–284. https://doi.org/10.1215/00182168-9653491

17. Velásquez Nimatuj IA. Struggles and obstacles in Indigenous women's fight for justice in Guatemala. July 29, 2016. Available at: https://sites.utexas.edu/llilas-benson-magazine/2016/07/29/struggles-and-obstacles-in-indigenous-womens-fight-for-justice-in-guatemala. Accessed December 7, 2023.

18. Casa de la Memoria: Kaji Tulam Guatemala. Virtual Exhibit. Available at: https://casadelamemoria.org.gt. Accessed February 16, 2024.

19. Benton A. On the Racial Immunologics of Humanitarian Organizations. SOAS University of London Humanitarianism Seminar Series, April 12, 2022. Available at: https://blogs.soas.ac.uk/humanitarian-hub/2022/04/12/global-health-on-the-racial-immunologics-of-humanitarian-organizations. Accessed March 12, 2024.

20. Kleinman A. Moral experience and ethical reflection: can ethnography reconcile them? A Quandary for "the new bioethics." *Daedalus* 1999;128(4):69–97.

Barriers to and Facilitators of Pediatric Vaccination Reporting in Four US States, 2023

Sara Israelsen-Hartley, MPP, and Nathan A. Boucher, DrPH, MS, MPA

In a 2023 sequential explanatory mixed-methods study in four US states, we identified barriers and facilitators experienced by Vaccines for Children (VFC) program providers in reporting vaccination data to state immunization information systems (IISs). We found the following: VFC providers value accurate, robust, and widely used IISs. IIS reporting is easier with but does not require an electronic health record. Negative interactions with IISs and VFC officials and limited practice capacity are barriers to reporting. The COVID-19 pandemic highlighted the need for a nationwide vaccination database. (*Am J Public Health*. 2024;114(6):569–574. https://doi.org/10.2105/AJPH.2024.307638)

AJPH June 2024, Vol. 114, No. 6

We share key findings from a sequential explanatory mixed-methods study to identify barriers to and facilitators of vaccination reporting from the perspective of pediatric Vaccines for Children (VFC) program providers, both before and during the COVID-19 pandemic.

STUDY OBJECTIVE

We sought to identify barriers and facilitators experienced by VFC program providers in reporting pediatric vaccinations to state immunization information systems (IISs)[1] before and during the COVID-19 pandemic, focusing on states where reporting was already required by state law or state VFC contract.

RESEARCH QUESTION

We asked what public health officials can do to reduce study-identified barriers and increase reporting to a state IIS among VFC providers.

PARTICIPANTS, SAMPLE GEOGRAPHIC LOCATION, SETTING, AND YEAR OF STUDY

We interviewed 23 professionals involved with vaccinating children as either a pediatrician, nurse, clinical assistant, or vaccination administrator across four states: Colorado, Connecticut, Maryland, and Massachusetts (Table A, available as a supplement to the online version of this article at http://www.ajph.org). Interviews spanned January to March 2023: Colorado (n = 5), Connecticut (n = 6), Maryland (n = 7), and Massachusetts (n = 5). These semistructured interviews ranged from 23 to 65 minutes, averaging 41.5 minutes.

METHODS

Our study used a sequential explanatory mixed-methods approach. We first reviewed the Centers for Disease Control and Prevention's IIS dashboard data quality reports for each state. Through multiple data-screening rounds, we narrowed our query to four states: Colorado, Connecticut, Maryland, and Massachusetts. These four states require that VFC providers report vaccinations to an IIS, either through state law (MD, MA, CT) or state VFC contract (CO). There is no federal law requiring IIS reporting, and thus many states do not require it.[2] These four states also experienced multiple years of less than 95% reporting rates yet saw improvement from 2019 to 2021, despite pandemic challenges.

Our multidisciplinary research team developed a semistructured interview guide following a literature review and informational telephone conversations with several vaccination leaders. The guide focused on three domains: (1) existing processes for vaccination data entry, (2) perceived barriers to and facilitators of vaccination entry, and (3) COVID-19 pandemic impacts. We then contacted 112 individuals, organizations, and practices by telephone, e-mail, or both, including American Academy of Pediatrics state chapters, professional medical organizations, public health offices, and private pediatric practices. Of the 112 contacts, 24 people agreed to a telephone interview, and 23 qualified for further conversations. We included only providers who vaccinated children, had at least four years of VFC participation, spoke English, and consented to a recorded interview.

We electronically recorded all interviews, transcribed them with Otter (Otter.ai, Inc., Mountain View, CA), and verified them for accuracy. We analyzed transcripts using a two-coder descriptive content analysis with an inductive approach.[3] We then completed analysis using NVivo version 12 (QSR International, Melbourne, Australia) for data management.[4] To develop themes from our codes, we relied on three sequential frameworks: barrier to or facilitator of optimal reporting; whether that barrier or facilitator was the result of people, processes, or technology[5]; and the level it occurred on, beginning at the individual and progressing through practice, peer providers, state level, and beyond, as shown in Table 1. The people, processes, and technology dimensions are key to organizational change and are well described in the information technology literature. Deficiencies in any of the three dimensions create barriers to organizational change.

KEY FINDINGS

We selected two main findings from our full results to discuss that refute an assumed barrier and highlight potentially underexplored facilitators: (1) personal connections and practice capacity shape interaction with IISs, and (2) provider willingness to enter historical vaccination data produces a more robust IIS yet is currently unincentivized.

Most health care providers rely on electronic health records (EHRs) to manage patient records.[6] However, high costs and maintenance requirements make EHRs less common in public health offices and federally qualified health centers—where many children receive vaccinations.

The majority of participants believed that not having an EHR would be a significant barrier to IIS reporting. Of the 23 providers interviewed, 5 (22%) did not have a formal EHR. Yet these five providers, who all worked in public health, reported vaccination data to the IIS either directly or through an IIS-provided interface. Four of the five had been doing so for years. The fifth provider's IIS participation began in 2020 as a result of a new state law. These providers said they enjoyed their state IIS and relied on it or an IIS interface to manage inventory, order vaccines, and generate reports as they would have used an EHR. This finding contradicts a prevailing notion that an EHR is required for IIS participation.

Regardless of EHR use, providers said interactions with IIS and VFC officials influenced their feelings about the VFC program and vaccination reporting. Some providers noted very negative interactions with VFC officials, which they felt were more punitive than problem solving. Providers believed this environment discouraged some providers from participating in the VFC program, potentially reducing IIS reporting.

In our first main finding, the specific barriers to and facilitators of vaccination reporting fit in the framework categories of people and technology: they involve human interactions as well as the presence or lack of an electronic system. They occur on levels 2 and 4: practice and state IIS and VFC officials, as they deal with office-level resources and relationships with state administrators.

The four states we studied each require that providers report data to the IISs for currently administered vaccinations; however, there is no requirement to enter historical vaccinations. Despite this, nearly all providers said patients often present paper records showing (1) a vaccination received years ago, (2) a vaccination received recently from an out-of-state provider, or (3) a vaccination received recently from an in-state provider not reporting to the IIS. This last situation was especially common during early mass COVID-19 vaccination clinics. Providers then had the option to add historical vaccinations to a patient's file—either through their EHR or to the IIS directly.

This extra step requires time and staffing availability, which is often in short supply.[7] Providers in smaller public health offices are often the only people handling vaccinations and sometimes feel overwhelmed. For these providers especially, complying with real-time documentation laws takes precedence over entering historical data. This may be an occasional barrier to IIS entry; however, most providers said they enter historical data because they believe a more accurate IIS helps them better care for their patients.

The COVID-19 pandemic greatly increased how often providers entered historical data. This is because the country lacks a nationwide vaccination database, which prevents providers from easily accessing records of patients who moved from another state or who live in one state but seek care in another. Nearly every provider expressed frustration with this gap. (See additional provider quotations in

TABLE 1— Barriers to IIS Reporting Among VFC Providers

Barrier	People	Process	Technology
Level 1: Barriers at the individual level	I am the only one in my office who handles vaccination reporting.	I'm going to retire soon, no need to change now.	I have a hard time learning new things about technology from technology.
	I am uncomfortable with technology.	I never received any training on how to do vaccination reporting.	I keep forgetting my password, I always need to set a new password.
	Too many people in my office need my help navigating the IIS; it's overwhelming.	I don't see how this helps our practice.	I don't have my own IIS login.
		This seems like more work than it's worth.	I can't find the patient or patient records I seek.
		I don't have time for training.	I can't generate the reports I want.
		We gave so many COVID-19 shots, sometimes I struggled to manually enter in that data.	If there's a technical glitch, I often have to reenter data and that's frustrating.
Level 2: Barriers at the practice level	We are short staffed.	We have always done vaccination entry on paper, why change?	Our Internet is not reliable.
	There is only one person with an IIS login in our office.	We are not patients' primary care home and may only see them one time.	Our office doesn't have an IT department to help with technical problems.
	Our immunization nurse doesn't like technology.	We are a small office and don't do many pediatric vaccinations or we are giving fewer vaccinations than we have in the past.	Our EHR vendor doesn't seem to be interested in making our system better.
		We don't spend time on IIS training at work.	Our EHR doesn't interface well with the state IIS.
		Mass vaccination clinics were overwhelming; we couldn't keep up with data entry.	We struggle to reconcile our vaccination records with the IIS.
Level 3: Barriers at the peer provider level (in-state)	Some providers still don't understand they should report.	There is no clear or consistent message on who should be reporting and what data to report.	My EHR can't get data from other providers if they don't use the IIS.
	Sometimes other providers won't share information about a shared patient.	Our state law doesn't have or doesn't enforce consequences for providers who don't report.	
	If school nurses can't access the IIS, it's hard to share vaccination data.	There's not an easy way to tell other providers about errors I see coming from their office.	
	Some providers enter data incorrectly to the IIS.	Some providers don't use the IIS, especially pharmacies and urgent cares.	
Level 4: Barriers at the state IIS and VFC official level	I don't know who to call with questions.	The VFC recertification process is onerous.	The online training videos are not helpful.
	The IIS staff isn't available when I have questions.	The VFC process is costly, especially if we need a new refrigerator, etc.	The IIS interface isn't working correctly.
	The IIS staff can't answer my questions.	The VFC process is frustrating and affects how I feel about the IIS.	The IIS itself isn't working correctly.
	It seems like the VFC staff is more interested in enforcing rules than helping me solve problems.	We are still waiting for the state IIS team to help connect our EHR to the IIS.	The IIS is not a seamless match with our EHRs.
			The IIS has duplicate records for the same patient and struggles with records for twins.
			I can't fix the IIS errors I find.
			The bidirectional flow of data isn't working.
			I can't print records directly or easily from the IIS.
			My upload to the IIS isn't immediate.

Continued

TABLE 1— Continued

Barrier	People	Process	Technology
Level 5: Barriers at the general public level	Parents don't want their child's vaccination records in the IIS so they opt out.	There's no official policy or process in our office for entering historical vaccination data.	There is no nationwide patient identification number for easy transfer of healthcare data between providers.
	Parents provide incorrect information about their child's vaccination history.	There is no political will in my state to draft any laws related to vaccination or vaccination data reporting.	There is no nationwide IIS.
Level 6: Barriers at the peer provider level (out-of-state)	Sometimes other providers won't share information about a shared patient.		Our IIS doesn't connect to any other states, or we connect to only a few states.

Note. EHR = electronic health record; IIS = immunization information system; VFC = Vaccines for Children program.

the Additional Results section of the Appendix, available as a supplement to the online version of this article at http://www.ajph.org.)

In our second main finding, the barriers to and facilitators of vaccination reporting encompass all three framework categories: people, process, and technology. They involve human capacity, required and optional steps in a process, and the lack of a nationwide electronic database. They occur on levels 1, 2, 5, and 6: individual, practice, general public, and other providers out of state.

EVALUATION, TRANSFERABILITY, AND ADVERSE EFFECTS

We sought to identify barriers to IIS reporting, and we present ideas for increasing IIS reporting among VFC providers. We found that a lack of an EHR is not a barrier to IIS reporting, but negative interactions with IIS and VFC staff are barriers. We also found that many providers take time to enter historical vaccinations into the IIS to ensure a robust, useful record,[8] but such behavior is currently neither incentivized nor rewarded.

Increasing IIS reporting means both reducing barriers and increasing facilitators. Creating opportunities for positive, real-time interactions between VFC and IIS officials and providers could increase provider willingness to report. Laws requiring robust reporting and penalizing nonreporting may increase IIS participation yet also cause unintended consequences if there is no compensatory funding to alleviate staffing shortages. Alternatively, incentivizing reporting and publicly praising compliance may be a gentler way to shift provider behavior. Developing a robust data information exchange among the existing 64 registries would reduce provider frustration and boost IIS accuracy.

We conducted this study during the COVID-19 public health emergency when the federal government provided COVID-19 vaccines at no cost and Centers for Disease Control and Prevention required reporting within 24 hours.[9] The public health emergency expired on May 11, 2023.[10] As COVID-19 vaccinations become part of the routine vaccination landscape—minus federal subsidies and reporting requirements—we must understand that providers' reporting of COVID-19 and routine vaccinations might change.[11]

We focused on pediatric vaccination reporting; however, future studies should address what might encourage providers in states with reporting laws to manually enter adults' historical vaccination records into their IISs (see Table B, available as a supplement to the online version of this article at http://www.ajph.org).

SCALABILITY

These findings may be applicable to other settings because of the nature of our sample. We interviewed providers across four states but were studying participation in a medically standardized procedure (vaccination) across a fairly standardized nationwide program (VFC). Our findings may also reflect the experiences of providers who live in states beyond the four we studied but where state law or VFC contracts also require IIS reporting.[12] Thus, the resources we developed to identify barriers and facilitators may be useful to a broader audience (Figure 1; Figure A, available as a supplement to the online version of this article at http://www.ajph.org). However, we also note that providers who did not return our calls might have shared different insights than those who agreed to interviews.

PUBLIC HEALTH SIGNIFICANCE

Vaccination remains one of the most impactful human discoveries of the

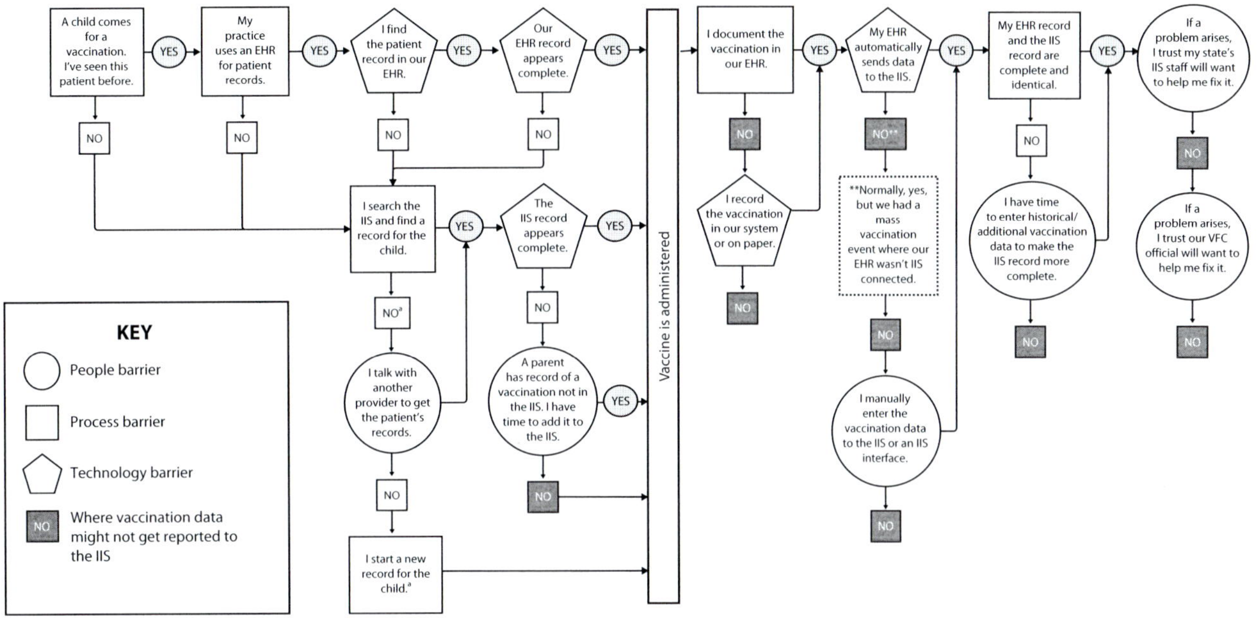

FIGURE 1— **Process Map of Which Barriers Stop Vaccination Data From Entering an Immunization Information System (IIS)**

Note. EHR = electronic health record; VFC = Vaccines for Children program.
[a]Misspelled names, especially hyphenated last names, or wrong birthdates can lead to difficulty finding a record or multiple records being created for the same patient.

past few centuries. The VFC program, which celebrated its 30th anniversary in 2023, ensures that all children can receive life-saving vaccines regardless of financial constraints.[13] Yet, state immunization information databases, which document these crucial doses, are not as accurate or complete as they could be.[14] This is because of negative interactions with IIS and VFC staff, provider constraints, and technological limitations. These barriers reduce the accuracy of IIS databases, affecting their usefulness for routine surveillance and emergency response.

The COVID-19 pandemic highlighted the need for accurate, real-time IIS participation, which our study found can happen with or without an EHR. Additionally, we learned that most providers participate in IIS data entry because they see their IIS as a tool to help them provide quality care. However, there is room for improvement.[15] Public health officials at both the jurisdiction and federal levels should consider ways to increase access to positive, real-time technical support, work toward interstate data sharing, and incentivize historical vaccination entry. These efforts will increase the robustness of IIS databases and help ensure ongoing provider participation. AJPH

ABOUT THE AUTHORS

At the time of the study, Sara Israelsen-Hartley was a master of public policy student, Sanford School of Public Policy, Duke University, Durham, NC. Nathan A. Boucher is an associate professor, Sanford School of Public Policy, Nursing School, and School of Medicine, Duke University.

CORRESPONDENCE

Correspondence should be sent to Sara Israelsen-Hartley, Sanford School of Public Policy, Box 90312, Durham, NC 27708 (e-mail: saraizzy@gmail.com). Reprints can be ordered at http://www.ajph.org by clicking the "Reprints" link.

PUBLICATION INFORMATION

Full Citation: Israelsen-Hartley S, Boucher NA. Barriers to and facilitators of pediatric vaccination reporting in four US states, 2023. *Am J Public Health*. 2024;114(6):569–574.

Acceptance Date: February 17, 2024.

DOI: https://doi.org/10.2105/AJPH.2024.307638

CONTRIBUTORS

S. Israelsen-Hartley reviewed and analyzed the Centers for Disease Control and Prevention data, recruited participants, conducted all interviews, led the qualitative data analysis, and wrote the first draft of the article. N. A. Boucher assisted with the development of the codebook and initial coding, suggested improvements to the analysis, and provided feedback on the article. Both authors designed the study.

CONFLICTS OF INTEREST

The authors have no potential or actual conflicts of interest to disclose.

HUMAN PARTICIPANT PROTECTION

The Duke University institutional review board approved this study (IRB protocol no. 2023-0246).

REFERENCES

1. Hackell JM, Palevsky SL, Resnick M. Immunization information systems. *Pediatrics*. 2022;150(4): e2022059281. https://doi.org/10.1542/peds.2022-059281

2. Martin DW, Lowery NE, Brand B, Gold R, Horlick G. Immunization information systems: a decade of progress in law and policy. *J Public Health Manag Pract.* 2015;21(3):296–303. https://doi.org/10.1097/PHH.0000000000000040
3. Vaismoradi M, Turunen H, Bondas T. Content analysis and thematic analysis: implications for conducting a qualitative descriptive study. *Nurs Health Sci.* 2013;15(3):398–405. https://doi.org/10.1111/nhs.12048
4. Saldaña J. *The Coding Manual for Qualitative Researchers.* 2nd ed. SAGE; 2013.
5. Shea CM, Malone R, Weinberger M, et al. Assessing organizational capacity for achieving meaningful use of electronic health records. *Health Care Manage Rev.* 2014;39(2):124–133. https://doi.org/10.1097/HMR.0b013e3182860937
6. Office of the National Coordinator for Health Information Technology. Office-based physician electronic health record adoption. Available at: https://www.healthit.gov/data/quickstats/office-based-physician-electronic-health-record-adoption. Accessed April 11, 2023.
7. Zhavoronkova M, Custer BD, Neal A. How to ease the nursing shortage in America. May 23, 2022. Available at: https://www.americanprogress.org/article/how-to-ease-the-nursing-shortage-in-america. Accessed April 3, 2023.
8. Groom H, Hopkins DP, Pabst LJ, et al. Immunization information systems to increase vaccination rates: a community guide systematic review. *J Public Health Manag Pract.* 2015;21(3):227–248. https://doi.org/10.1097/PHH.0000000000000069
9. Centers for Disease Control and Prevention. COVID-19 vaccination program jurisdiction operations interim operational guidance. October 29, 2020. Available at: https://www.cdc.gov/vaccines/imz-managers/downloads/Covid-19-Vaccination-Program-Interim_Playbook.pdf. Accessed February 3, 2023.
10. US Department of Health and Human Services. Fact sheet: end of the COVID-19 public health emergency. May 9, 2023. Available at: https://www.hhs.gov/about/news/2023/05/09/fact-sheet-end-of-the-covid-19-public-health-emergency.html. Accessed October 18, 2023.
11. Santoki A, Boucher N. Investigating barriers to vaccination among Durham County's vulnerable populations. *N C Med J.* 2021;82(3):164–170. https://doi.org/10.18043/ncm.82.3.164
12. Centers for Disease Control and Prevention. Immunization Information Systems (IIS) dashboard. Available at: https://wwwn.cdc.gov/IISDashboard/Query.aspx. Accessed April 12, 2023.
13. Centers for Disease Control and Prevention. Benefits from immunization during the Vaccines for Children program era—United States, 1994–2013. *MMWR Morb Mortal Wkly Rep.* 2014;63(16):352–355.
14. Scharf LG, Coyle R, Adeniyi K, et al. Current challenges and future possibilities for immunization information systems. *Acad Pediatr.* 2021;21(4 suppl):S57–S64. https://doi.org/10.1016/j.acap.2020.11.008
15. Benjamin-Chung J, Reingold A. Measuring the success of the US COVID-19 vaccine campaign—it's time to invest in and strengthen immunization information systems. *Am J Public Health.* 2021;111(6):1078–1080. https://doi.org/10.2105/AJPH.2021.306177

On Detecting Endemicity: Insights from All-Cause Mortality Patterns During Epidemic Transitions

Jeremy Samuel Faust, MS, MD

ABOUT THE AUTHOR

Jeremy Samuel Faust is with the Department of Emergency Medicine, Mass General Brigham and the Division of Health Services Research, Harvard Medical School, Boston.

See also Excess Mortality Calculations: Methods and Uses, pp. 580–609.

During epidemic outbreaks, transitions to endemicity are often discussed, but rarely, if ever, defined. Analyzing all-cause mortality patterns may be useful.

As Vandenbroucke and Pearce write in this issue of *AJPH* (p. 593), all-cause excess mortality—rates exceeding expected values, agnostic to cause—provides perhaps the best and least biased measure of the most severe effects of an acute outbreak.

And yet, in the fullness of time, there is no such thing as an excess death, as all people die precisely once. These observations are not contradictions. Rather, they present an opportunity to understand features of a recent epidemic, and to aid in the detection of either the endemic phase of an outbreak, or the eradication of the novel threat. Here, I will discuss how by considering specific patterns of all-cause mortality, it can be determined when a pathogen has likely become endemic. In addition, these patterns can reveal important information about the cohort of excess decedents.

FACTORS IN ALL-CAUSE MORTALITY SUPPORTING ENDEMICITY

Several mortality-related measures can help determine if an endemic phase has been reached. While no single metric is definitive, the presence of one or more points toward endemicity:

1. The recoupling of observed and expected deaths. In an amply sized population, the correlations (weekly or monthly) between observed and expected deaths are reliably strong (Figure 1a, years 0–2). Acute outbreaks marked by sudden increases in mortality uncouple these correlations (Figure 1a, years 2–4). Endemicity is supported when recoupling of observed and expected deaths occurs (Figure 1a, years 4–7).
2. The resumption of typical mortality shares across demographics. Generally, the shares of all-cause mortality by age, sex, race/ethnicity, etc., are disparate, but stable. Outbreaks disrupt these norms. The return to preoutbreak mortality share patterns (including regrettable disparities) supports endemicity.
3. The resumption of typical variability across jurisdictions. Typically, variance in mortality by jurisdiction is stable. Outbreaks widen mortality dispersion across jurisdictions, as pathogens move through various regions. A return to preoutbreak variance, therefore, supports endemicity.
4. If novel pathogen-attributed deaths rise during times of increased disease incidence, but all-cause mortality does not, endemicity is supported (assuming decreases in other causes of deaths have not offset pathogen-driven increases).

CESSATION OF EXCESS MORTALITY MAY NOT SUPPORT ENDEMICITY

Initially, I believed that the cessation of all-cause excess mortality or the appearance of deficit mortality might indicate endemicity. However, I wish to highlight that this may not always be so. Following an outbreak, three conditions may occur: all-cause excess mortality cessation, the appearance of deficit mortality, or chronic (though reduced) excess mortality (Figure 1a; years 4–7, scenarios B, C, and A, respectively). None of these conditions inherently supports endemicity, but instead, may carry information about the pandemic decedents (Figure 1b, Figure 2). Indeed, each of the three scenarios can occur absent the recoupling of observed and expected deaths, the resumption of usual expected shares, or

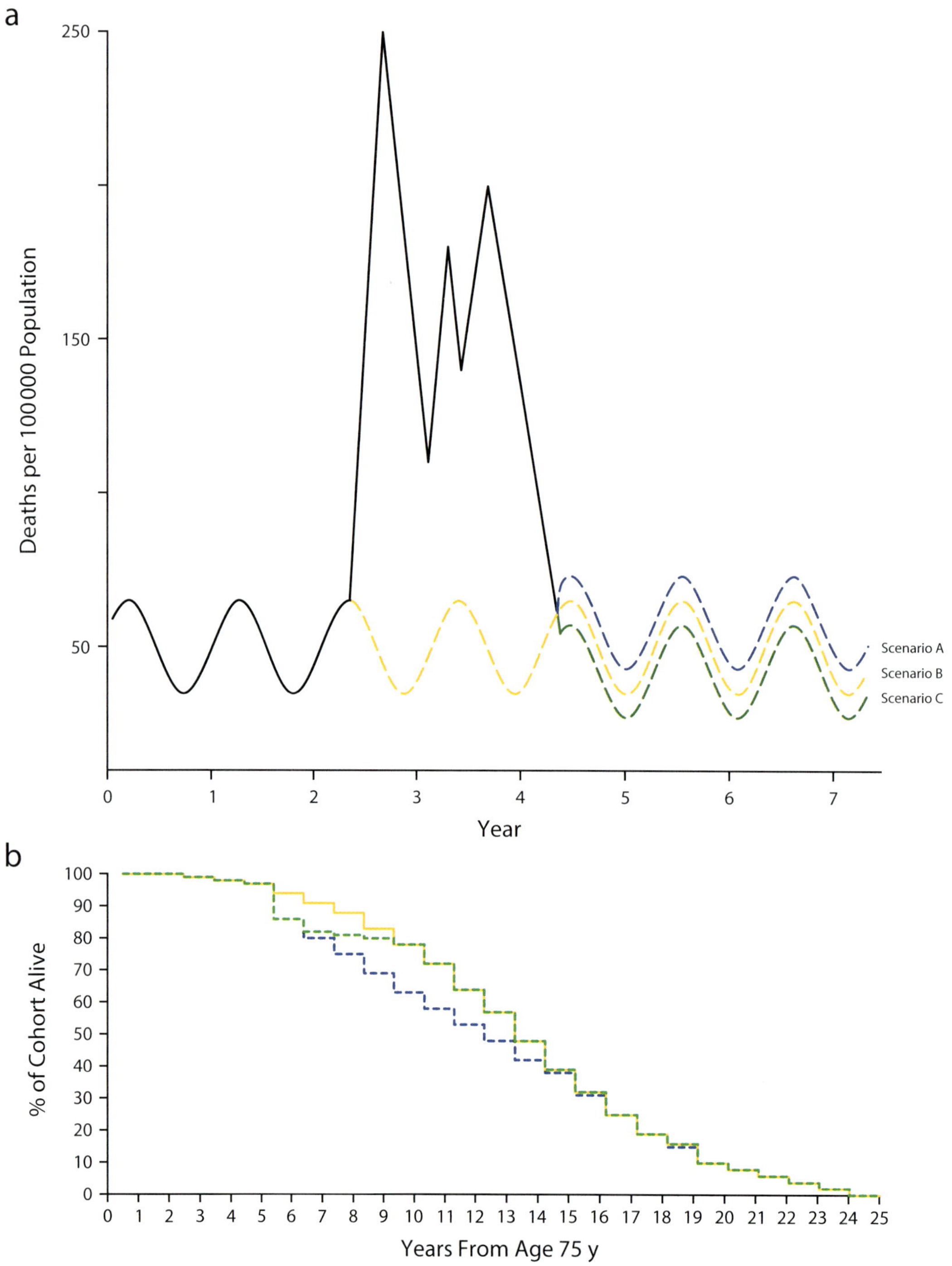

FIGURE 1— Mortality Dynamics Before, During, and After a Pandemic by (a) Observed and Expected Mortality Scenarios and (b) Different Mortality Scenarios

Note. Part a displays a hypothetical time series of mortality data over a 7-year period. The solid black line represents the observed mortality rate before a pandemic (years 0–2) and during a pandemic (years 2–4), The yellow dashed line shows the expected mortality rate in the absence of the pandemic (i.e., counterfactual mortality) starting in year 2. Starting in year 4, three postoutbreak scenarios are shown. Scenario A represents a chronic increase above expected mortality while scenario C represents a chronic decrease ("deficit mortality") during the postacute phase of the outbreak. Scenario B represents a continuation of prepandemic expected mortality. Part b depicts a Kaplan-Meier survival curve under different scenarios. The yellow solid line symbolizes the original Kaplan-Meier survival curve (no outbreak). The green dashed line shows a scenario (similar to scenario C in part a) wherein a disproportionately greater increase in mortality occurred among individuals with lower life expectancies. The blue dash-dotted line depicts a scenario (similar to scenario A in part a) wherein a disproportionately greater increase in mortality occurred among those with higher life expectancies.

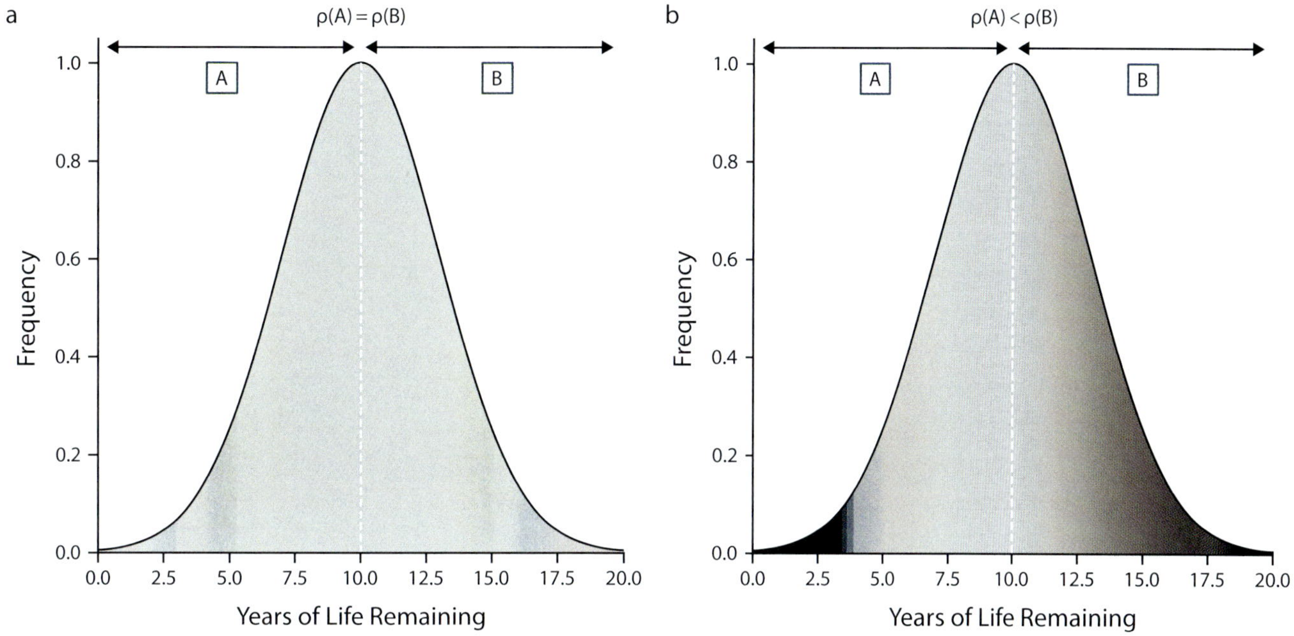

FIGURE 2— Pandemic Mortality Dynamics of a Cohort of 80-Year-Old Persons (a) Overall and (b) With Risk-Specific Pandemic-Associated All-Cause Mortality Odds Ratios Shown as Density Under the Curve

Note. Part a shows a normal distribution mortality curve. The mean life expectancy for the cohort is represented by the central white dashed vertical line. The density (ρ) of shading represents the relative contribution to increased mortality during an outbreak, across the life expectancy spectrum. The homogenous shading indicates that, in this instance, any changes in mortality are evenly distributed across the risk pool. Part b shows a similar curve as the left, but with altered relative contributions to increased mortality. In part b, the average density to the right of the mean (vertical dashed line) is greater than the density (ρ) to the left of the mean (despite the local area with the greatest density appearing at the far left).

typical variance ranges, as discussed. To understand why, let us consider the three postoutbreak conditions:

1. Excess mortality cessation (Figure 1a, scenario B). While appearing reassuring, if the epidemic disproportionately affected persons with shorter life expectancy, equilibrium has not been reached. Rather, revised rates of expected mortality should be lower than counterfactual expected rates. Therefore, the cessation of excess mortality (when observed deaths approximately matches expected deaths) might actually represent excess mortality, once pull-forward/healthy survivor effects have been considered.
2. The appearance of deficit mortality (Figure 1a, scenario C). After an outbreak, historically low death rates may appear. This, too, may be falsely reassuring. However, as above, if most excess decedents had short life expectancies, revised expected rates of postoutbreak mortality should be far lower. Therefore, what appears as deficit mortality might really be excess mortality.
3. The appearance of stable chronic excess mortality (Figure 1a, scenario A). The emergence of chronic excess mortality—i.e., low, relatively constant rates of excess mortality—is perhaps the most confusing possibility. (It also appears to be the condition we are seeing at this point in the COVID-19 experience.) While chronic excess mortality might seemingly argue against endemicity, continuous but relatively stable excess mortality can be consistent with endemicity (for reasons not dissimilar from those mentioned previously, though that may seem surprising). There are at least two possible explanations to consider. First, if the pathogen remains dangerous enough to the survivor cohort that it poses an ongoing (albeit lower) risk, chronic excess mortality may occur. That is, any pull-forward/healthy survivor effects are offset by the pathogen's continued presence. Second, chronic excess mortality can appear (despite outward appearances) when the mortality distribution density during the acute outbreak has, on average, been disproportionately concentrated among the healthier half of the population (Figure 2a; the curve shows homogeneous excess mortality across the risk spectrum compared

with Figure 2b, where changes are heterogeneous across the risk spectrum). This pattern would be observed if risks taken in the population correlated to perceived health except at the far left of the curve shown in Figure 2b; restated, healthier people (the right half of Figure 2b) experienced greater exposure to the pathogen (owing to higher risk tolerance) during the outbreak. However, persons with extremely high mortality risks (i.e., those with high risk of mortality during years 0–3) may have been unable to avoid pathogen exposure; for example, persons living in long-term care facilities, or those who require frequent medical visits. This scenario could explain why nursing home residents experienced high mortality rates during the early COVID-19 outbreak, but today's survivor cohort may (seemingly paradoxically) actually be less healthy on average than the prepandemic population. If mortality rates on the far right of the graph were, say, 8-fold below the rates on the left (e.g., 1000 vs 8000 deaths per 100 000 population), but associated years of lost life were, on average, 10-fold greater (e.g., 15 years vs 1.5 years), the survivor population would have lower life expectancies. A scenario like this is rarely considered but seems likely.

ENDEMICITY VS ERADICATION

Without further analysis, conditions supporting endemicity might be indistinguishable from conditions consistent with eradication. However, if eradication has occurred, the Figure 1 scenario C and A curves should eventually merge with the scenario B curve (sooner in scenario C and later in scenario A, reflecting the differences in years of lost life per excess death). An equilibrium would only be reached once the area under the curve from the acute phase (Figure 1a, years 2–4) equals either the area between the curves of scenario A and B or the area between the curves of scenario B and C during the postacute phase. An alternative way to visualize this would be to observe a smaller-than-expected population after an outbreak (Figure 1b) returning to normal levels either four years (pull-forward effect) or 11 years later.

Meanwhile, in scenario B, distinguishing between eradication and an endemic threat that has essentially been neutralized (by immunity or treatments that abolish mortality) is challenging. Combining these observations with viral surveillance (e.g., wastewater monitoring), however, would be definitive.

Alternatively, if a pathogen has become endemic (marked by low but persistently elevated mortality), the curves of scenarios A and C would never merge with that of scenario B. Here, the life expectancy of the survivor cohort would eventually be found to have increased (scenario C) or decreased (scenario A) compared with the preoutbreak era population.

CONTEXTUALIZING EXPECTED DEATHS (THE "NULL VALUE")

The general usefulness of excess mortality turns on the reliability and interpretation of expected deaths (the "null value"). Let us explore this during the three outbreak phases:

1. Prior to outbreaks, long-term analyses of observed deaths define the bounds of predictability. Identifying how much variance (including seasonal variation) exists at baseline can help epidemic teams determine if the magnitude of a sudden mortality increase is cause for concern—that is, local thresholds that divide signal and noise. Is a weekly increase over expected deaths of 2% meaningful? Is 10%? Models can easily determine thresholds for mortality that are two, three, or many standard deviations above historical means. These thresholds depend on the population size, baseline mortality rates, and the general stability of preoutbreak conditions. The study of preoutbreak all-cause mortality, therefore, can establish thresholds useful for threat detection (adjusted for lag, if needed). While this work was not common before COVID-19, the rapid assembly of models identified that sudden increases in all-cause mortality that accompanied the initial outbreaks were massive outliers.
2. During outbreaks, knowing the number of expected deaths permits context (i.e., a counterfactual) for the number of recorded deaths. This allows an assessment of the magnitude of the problem. Nor is lag an insurmountable obstacle for using all-cause mortality this way. In Massachusetts, more than 98% of weekly deaths are routinely known to the Registry of Vital Statistics (and its partners) within three days of the previous week.
3. After outbreaks. The return to mortality rates similar to preoutbreak levels can, as mentioned previously, be helpful in determining characteristics of the endemic phase and the survivor cohort.

OTHER OBSERVATIONS REGARDING EXCESS MORTALITY

When considering excess mortality, unit choices are often overlooked. For instance, the number of excess deaths may seem small in populations with low baseline mortality rates, which may obscure important implications. For example, if mortality among a cohort of 30-year-old persons increases by 40% (from 100 to 140 among 100 000 people), only 40 excess deaths would be measured. However, assuming a life expectancy of 80 years, the years of lost life would amount to 2000. Meanwhile, a 10% increase among a cohort of 80-year-old persons (from 1000–1100 per 100 000) with prior life expectancies of eight years would result in 100 excess deaths, but only 800 years of lost life. Generally, the lower the baseline mortality rate, the greater the years of lost life. Deciding whether to report the number of excess deaths, rate (per capita), or observed-to-expected ratio dramatically influences the insights; these metrics have distinct meanings.

Additionally, while age standardization is useful in comparing outcomes across jurisdiction, the practice obscures ground conditions. Age-stratification may be more appropriate. For example, a region with many older persons might need to take greater precautions during outbreaks. Age standardization can give the false impression that such a region performed "as well" as one with a younger population, when, in fact, that was not so. Choices regarding measurement and reporting should be made carefully.

CONCLUSIONS: EMBRACING A CONTRADICTION

While excess deaths may not, in the final analysis, truly exist, early deaths do. Indeed, 99.9% of those who died of 1918 H1N1 would be dead by now anyway. Nevertheless, the tens of millions who perished in 1918 to 1919 were deprived of unrecoverable years of lost life.

Herein, I have proposed a paradigm for the detection of the endemic phase of an outbreak with respect to mortality. However, endemicity has different meanings. Declaring a pathogen endemic with respect to mortality alone does not imply that morbidity has been neutralized. Furthermore, endemicity may prove transient, especially with a rapidly mutating virus. Still, without a specific framework, there is the risk that subjective declarations of endemicity will be made once we are exhausted of a pathogen, but well before it has exhausted its most profound effects upon us. AJPH

CORRESPONDENCE

Correspondence should be sent to Jeremy Samuel Faust, 10 Vining Street, Boston, MA 02115 (e-mail: Jsfaust@bwh.harvard.edu). Reprints can be ordered at http://www.ajph.org by clicking the "Reprints" link.

PUBLICATION INFORMATION

Full Citation: Faust JS. On detecting endemicity: insights from all-cause mortality patterns during epidemic transitions. *Am J Public Health*. 2024;114(6):575–579.

Acceptance Date: March 26, 2024.

DOI: https://doi.org/10.2105/AJPH.2024.307678

ACKNOWLEDGMENTS

I wish to thank Harlan Krumholz and the team at the Yale Center for Outcomes Research and Evaluation, as well as Benjamin Renton. But for our ongoing collaboration in the study of excess mortality, this work would not be possible. I would also like to acknowledge Benjamin Renton and Alexander Junxiang Chen for assisting in formatting the figures.

CONFLICTS OF INTEREST

The author has no conflicts of interest to disclose.

Malignant Neglect: Accounting for Public Disinterest in Deteriorating Health Outcomes in the United States

Steven H. Woolf, MD, MPH

ABOUT THE AUTHOR

Steven H. Woolf is with the Center on Society and Health and Department of Family Medicine, Virginia Commonwealth University School of Medicine, Richmond, VA.

See also Excess Mortality Calculations: Methods and Uses, pp. 575–609.

AJPH June 2024, Vol. 114, No. 6

In this issue, Vandenbroucke and Pearce (p. 593) discuss technical issues surrounding the measurement of excess deaths during the COVID-19 pandemic. Excess deaths refers to the difference between observed deaths and the number expected under ordinary circumstances. The United States experienced a higher rate of excess deaths than most developed countries, suggesting that deficiencies in the US pandemic response caused needless deaths.[1]

Long before the pandemic, expert panels were documenting a US health disadvantage relative to other countries. Studies documented a widening gap between life expectancy in the United States and in peer countries (Figure 1). For decades, US mortality rates for many causes of death—and the prevalence of risk factors ranging from obesity to firearm ownership—have consistently been higher than in other high-income countries.[2] The resulting death toll has been enormous. Between 1980 and 2019, an estimated 11 million US deaths would have been averted had the United States experienced the mortality rates of other wealthy nations.[3]

Evidence of deteriorating health among Americans is mounting. US life expectancy plateaued after 2010, a trend attributed to rising mortality rates in the working-age population (ages 25–64 years). Contributing factors included drug overdoses, alcohol-related conditions, suicide, and cardiometabolic disease.[4] All-cause mortality in the pediatric population (ages 1–19 years) began increasing in 2020, meaning that children are now less likely to reach adulthood. Factors contributing to the increase include suicide and homicide (mostly involving firearms), as well as drug overdoses and motor vehicle crashes.[5]

Socioeconomic and racial inequities add to the death toll in the United States. Galea et al. estimated that approximately 240 000 deaths would have been averted in one year alone if US adults with low education experienced the mortality rates of those with higher education.[6] Another study estimated that more than 880 000 deaths would have been averted over the course of a decade if the non-Hispanic Black population experienced the mortality rates of the non-Hispanic White population.[7] A recent study estimated that racial/ethnic health inequities cost the nation more than $400 billion—in 2018 alone.[8]

The larger question about this literature, which sounds the alarm about deteriorating US health outcomes, is whether anyone is listening. Although such research is consumed by epidemiologists and public health experts, there is little evidence that the lay public or policymakers are aware of this crisis, let alone acting on it.[9] "Malignant neglect"[10] prevails. The statistics accumulate year after year, but little is done to address the root causes responsible for excess deaths.

This complacency could have at least six explanations. First, the public may be unaware that a crisis exists. Alarming studies generate occasional news coverage, but the media quickly move onto the next story. Public officials say little about the topic. Few politicians discuss rising death rates or raise concerns that the health and longevity of Americans have fallen far behind other countries. There was little outcry from parents when researchers reported rising death rates among US children.

Second, people may know the research but not sense a crisis. A decline in life expectancy from 79 to 78 years may seem inconsequential to laypeople, a detail they assume should concern only the elderly. They may not realize that the current decrease in US life expectancy signals thousands of premature deaths among young and

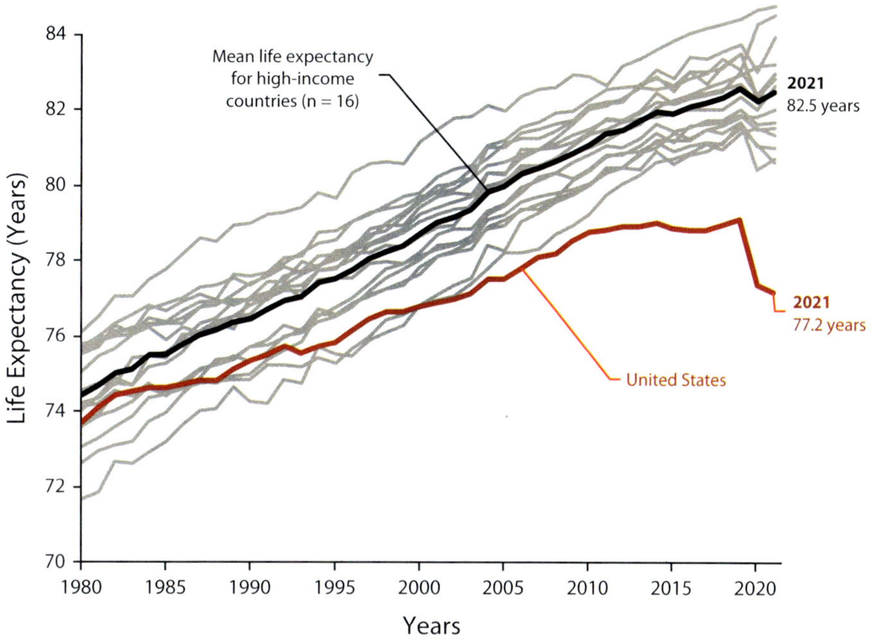

FIGURE 1— Life Expectancy in the United States and Other High-Income Countries, 1980–2021

Note. Gray lines plot life expectancy for 16 comparison countries (Australia, Austria, Canada, Denmark, Finland, France, Germany, Italy, Japan, Netherlands, Norway, Portugal, Spain, Sweden, Switzerland, and the United Kingdom). Black line designates the average life expectancy of the 16 countries. Red line plots US life expectancy.

Source. Data obtained from United Nations, Department of Economic and Social Affairs, Population Division. World Population Prospects 2022: Data Sources. Available at: https://population.un.org/wpp/Download/Files/4_Metadata/WPP2022_Data_Sources.pdf. Accessed November 11, 2022.

middle-aged adults, cut down in the prime of their lives.[4] Rising mortality rates pose an existential crisis, but it may get lost in a sea of existential crises. A public inured to apocalyptic predictions about climate change, wars, and the collapse of democracy may pay little mind to unfavorable health statistics.

The evidence for a crisis may be unconvincing. A public accustomed to conflicting health research may assume that a paper reporting millions of excess deaths is only one scientist's interpretation of statistics, soon to be refuted by another. Skepticism about science has reached new heights. Facts are of waning importance, especially when they clash with strongly held beliefs. For example, evidence that dozens of countries have outperformed the United States might clash with populist beliefs in American exceptionalism.[11]

Third, the public may assume that the crisis concerns only other people, such as the poor or people of color. In an argument with racist overtones, they may believe that unfavorable national health statistics reflect the influence of criminal gangs or gritty neighborhoods they try to avoid, not realizing that the root causes also reside in their own homes. Although marginalized Americans do experience disproportionately high death rates, advantaged populations (e.g., White, wealthy, or insured Americans) also die earlier than their counterparts in other countries.[2] The US health disadvantage is systemic, affecting all groups.

Fourth, some may blame the crisis on a unitary cause, mistakenly believing that resolving that single issue will restore the health of Americans. The problem, they argue, is obesity, the environment, opioids, guns, or the health care system. All of these certainly contribute, but the roots of the US health disadvantage are upstream, systemic factors such as socioeconomic inequality, public policy, social values, and systemic racism.[2]

Fifth, many people may feel paralyzed to act because they are overwhelmed by the scale of the crisis, especially by calls to address the root causes or enact sweeping societal changes for problems that seem too large to solve. They may not realize that many solutions are policies already on the table—on current ballot initiatives and in campaign speeches—such as creating middle-class jobs, investing in education, expanding affordable housing, and enacting minimum wage or paid leave policies.

Finally, other priorities may supersede the desire for good health. Health is the foremost concern among health professionals, but not necessarily among everyone else. In polls, Americans rank health care—but not health itself—among their top concerns. Distant threats to health, decades hence, may seem less urgent than paying the bills and holding down jobs. Some people cherish their lifestyle over longevity. Often for ideological reasons, they may be willing to risk disease and injury rather than restrict their freedom to live as they wish. For example, warnings about the effect on life expectancy are unlikely to win over fervent gun owners.

Policies that have enabled other countries to achieve better health outcomes, especially those involving social welfare programs, are often resisted in the United States on political or ideological grounds, among them the fear of higher taxes or socialism. Powerful corporations and their shareholders have their own concerns. They oppose regulations that would interfere with business operations or cut into profits, even if they could save lives. Elected officials also have competing priorities, such as fiscal concerns and political agendas. Policies that would benefit population health often fall victim to the politician's drive to retain power and get reelected. Health-promoting measures that displease special interests are often nonstarters in political circles.

Research to document excess deaths in the United States remains vital, but equally important is research on how to communicate the findings in ways that engage the public and policymakers. The public health community is only beginning to apply (or teach) the principles of communication science, which for decades have enabled advertisers, media outlets, and social movements to manipulate public consciousness and behavior. Decisive efforts to improve health are unlikely until progress occurs in alerting Americans to crises and motivating them to act. AJPH

CORRESPONDENCE

Correspondence should be sent to Steven H. Woolf, MD, MPH, Center on Society and Health, Virginia Commonwealth University School of Medicine, 830 East Main St, Suite 5035, Richmond, VA 23298-0212 (e-mail: steven.woolf@vcuhealth.org). Reprints can be ordered at http://www.ajph.org by clicking the "Reprints" link.

PUBLICATION INFORMATION

Full Citation: Woolf SH. Malignant neglect: accounting for public disinterest in deteriorating health outcomes in the United States. *Am J Public Health*. 2024;114(6):580–582.

Acceptance Date: February 9, 2024.

DOI: https://doi.org/10.2105/AJPH.2024.307626

ORCID iD:

Steven H. Woolf https://orcid.org/0000-0001-9384-033X

ACKNOWLEDGMENTS

S. H. Woolf received partial funding from the National Center for Advancing Translational Sciences (grant UM1TR004360).

CONFLICTS OF INTEREST

The author has no conflicts of interest to report.

REFERENCES

1. Bilinski A, Thompson K, Emanuel E. COVID-19 and excess all-cause mortality in the US and 20 comparison countries, June 2021–March 2022. *JAMA*. 2023;329(1):92–94. https://doi.org/10.1001/jama.2022.21795
2. National Research Council, Institute of Medicine. *US Health in International Perspective: Shorter Lives, Poorer Health*. Woolf SH, Aron L, eds. Washington, DC: National Academies Press; 2013.
3. Bor J, Stokes AC, Raifman J, et al. Missing Americans: early death in the United States—1933–2021. *PNAS Nexus*. 2023;2(6):pgad173.
4. National Academies of Sciences, Engineering, and Medicine; Division of Behavioral and Social Sciences and Education; Committee on National Statistics; Committee on Population; Committee on Rising Midlife Mortality Rates and Socioeconomic Disparities. *High and Rising Mortality Rates Among Working-Age Adults*. Becker T, Majmundar MK, Harris KM, eds. Washington, DC: National Academies Press; 2021.
5. Woolf SH, Wolf ER, Rivara FP. The new crisis of increasing all-cause mortality in US children and adolescents. *JAMA*. 2023;329(12):975–976. https://doi.org/10.1001/jama.2023.3517
6. Galea S, Tracy M, Hoggatt KJ, Dimaggio C, Karpati A. Estimated deaths attributable to social factors in the United States. *Am J Public Health*. 2011;101(8):1456–1465. https://doi.org/10.2105/AJPH.2010.300086
7. Woolf SH, Johnson RE, Fryer GE Jr, Rust G, Satcher D. The health impact of resolving racial disparities: an analysis of US mortality data. *Am J Public Health*. 2004;94(12):2078–2081. https://doi.org/10.2105/AJPH.94.12.2078
8. LaVeist TA, Pérez-Stable EJ, Richard P, et al. The economic burden of racial, ethnic, and educational health inequities in the US. *JAMA*. 2023;329(19):1682–1692. https://doi.org/10.1001/jama.2023.5965
9. Diamond D. America has a life expectancy crisis. But it's not a political priority. *Washington Post*. December 28, 2023. Available at: https://www.washingtonpost.com/health/2023/12/28/life-expectancy-no-political-response. Accessed March 7, 2024.
10. Stuckler D, Basu S. Malignant neglect: the failure to address the need to prevent premature non-communicable disease morbidity and mortality. *PLoS Med*. 2013;10(6):e1001466. https://doi.org/10.1371/journal.pmed.1001466
11. Woolf SH. Falling behind: the growing gap in life expectancy between the United States and other countries, 1933–2021. *Am J Public Health*. 2023;113(9):970–980. https://doi.org/10.2105/AJPH.2023.307310

Excess Mortality as a Tool to Monitor the Evolution of Health Emergencies: Choices, Challenges, and Future Directions

Eugenio Paglino, MA, and Andrew C. Stokes, PhD

ABOUT THE AUTHORS

Eugenio Paglino is with the Population Studies Center, University of Pennsylvania, Philadelphia. Andrew C. Stokes is with the Boston University School of Public Health, Boston, MA.

See also Excess Mortality Calculations: Methods and Uses, pp. 575–609.

Excess mortality has become one of the most popular metrics to assess the impact of the COVID-19 pandemic across the world. Excess mortality has three key advantages relative to alternatives: (1) it requires relatively little data (in the most basic form, a historical time series of annual deaths), (2) it does not depend on whether causes of death are accurately assigned on death certificates, and (3) it can be compared across space and time.

EXCESS MORTALITY ESTIMATES AND THEIR INTERPRETATION

In this issue of *AJPH*, Vandenbroucke and Pearce (p. 593) discuss the many merits of the excess mortality metric and focus on its role as an inferential tool to compare the "performance" of different countries or subpopulations in containing the COVID-19 pandemic. As they note, this type of analysis is akin to a difference-in-differences design, albeit usually approached with less rigor than in the causal inference literature. The key assumption behind this approach is that there are no time-varying differences between the two units being compared (typically two countries). For example, differences in excess mortality in two countries would be informative about the effectiveness of the policies they implemented only if no other time-varying factor could explain them. Since policies are not randomly assigned and countries were on different mortality trajectories before the onset of the pandemic, the assumption of no time-varying differences is unlikely to hold in many comparisons. Vandenbroucke and Pearce reach the same conclusion and exhort researchers to more carefully discuss how the assumptions might be violated and how the violations would affect the interpretation of the results. We think that this discussion can be made more rigorous if five crucial choices are carefully considered.

DESIGNING AN EXCESS MORTALITY ANALYSIS

The first choice a researcher faces is how to estimate the number of deaths that would have been observed in the absence of the COVID-19 pandemic. The most basic method to obtain this counterfactual consists of averaging annual deaths over a number of prepandemic years. This approach, used by many early studies of excess mortality,[1] has the advantage of being simple. However, it ignores trends in mortality and population change; furthermore, unless combined with a statistical analysis, it does not lend itself to probabilistic statements on excess mortality. More robust methods consider linear and nonlinear time trends as well as seasonality, most commonly through either the inclusion of harmonics with varying periodicities[2] or with the use of seasonal[3] or nonseasonal autoregressive integrated moving average (ARIMA) models, and deliver both point estimates and uncertainty intervals for expected mortality. Typically, the more flexible approaches are attractive when few units are considered (e.g., national deaths stratified by age) but can become computationally challenging if applied to subnational geographic units.[4,5]

The second key choice faced by researchers is how many years to include in the baseline period on which the counterfactual is calibrated. When this decision has a substantial effect on the estimates, multiple options should be explored and the robustness of the analysis's key findings should be assessed.[6]

A third choice, also discussed by Vandenbroucke and Pearce, is whether to adjust for or stratify by important covariates, especially age. Whether such adjustments are needed or desirable depends on the amount of between-

AJPH June 2024, Vol. 114, No. 6

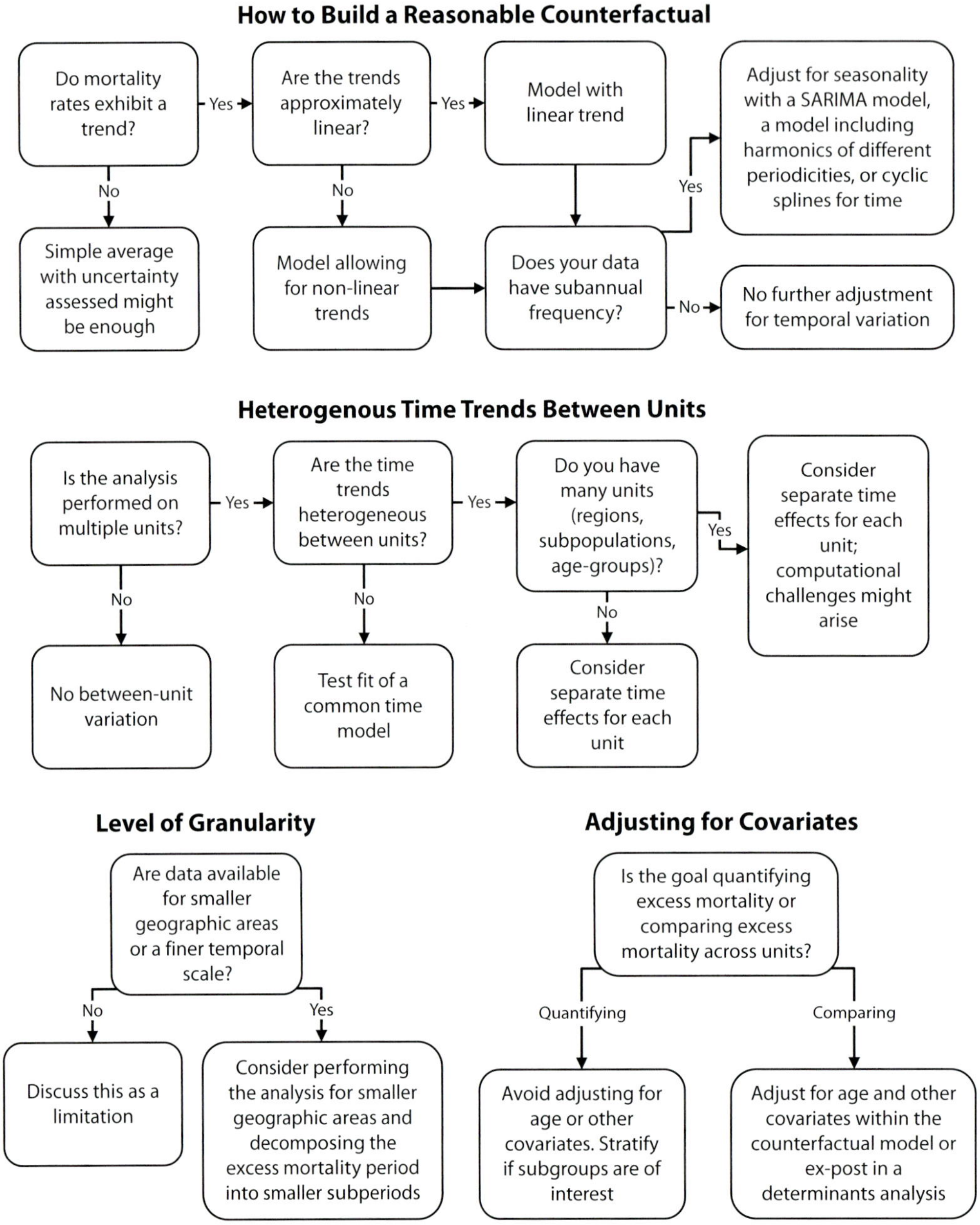

FIGURE 1— Key Factors to Consider When Estimating an Excess Mortality Model

Note. SARIMA = seasonal autoregressive integrated moving average. The figure illustrates the major choices and considerations that may be relevant to designing an excess mortality analysis, including how to construct a reasonable counterfactual, how to deal with potentially different time trends across units, which level of granularity to choose, and whether to adjust for covariates.

group heterogeneity and whether the principal aim is to conduct a causal analysis or descriptive study. In the first case, adjusting for potential confounders is crucial. However, in the second case, where description rather than causal inference is the goal, controlling for factors such as age and average income might be counterproductive as the estimates would no longer reflect the number of excess deaths that actually occurred. In such an instance, stratification may be a better approach as it allows for an examination of subgroup differences while maintaining the descriptive integrity of the estimates. For example, if excess mortality estimates are to be used to understand where to allocate recovery funds, we may prefer an estimate of the actual number of deaths that occurred (overall and across strata) rather than a synthetic estimate reflecting a hypothetical world in which all units shared similar characteristics.

A fourth choice is which level of spatial and temporal granularity to use. Regarding spatial units, national-level analyses have the advantage of fewer data requirements and offer appealing units for international comparisons. However, in countries where the spread of COVID-19 was geographically heterogeneous, national analyses might underestimate the impact of the pandemic. This limitation is particularly important when conducting cross-country or subnational comparisons and is closely related to the point made by Heuveline and Tzen that comparisons between small and densely populated areas (where virus transmission is easier) and large and sparsely populated ones (where the virus faces "natural" barriers) can be misleading.[7] A similar point can be made regarding temporal granularity. In countries, such as the United States, in which clear waves in COVID-19 and excess deaths have been documented,[5] yearly estimates might be unsatisfactory, especially when combined with a focus on national rather than subnational trends.

A fifth and final choice faced by researchers is which mortality indicator to present. Typical choices include crude excess death rates, age-standardized excess death rates, and age-specific excess death rates. Absolute counts of excess deaths, in total or by age, are also popular, together with relative excess presented as percentage or proportional increases in mortality. As pointed out by Vandenbroucke and Pearce, this choice should reflect assumptions about whether excess mortality would be additive (absolute measures would be more appropriate for comparisons) or multiplicative (relative measures would be more appropriate for comparisons). Another important consideration should be how interpretable different measures are. In general, we have found relative measures to have an advantage in this dimension as they do not require demographic knowledge to be interpreted. The key choices for modeling excess mortality are summarized in Figure 1.

EXCESS MORTALITY BEYOND THE COVID-19 PANDEMIC

While excess mortality analyses have become popular in the public health community during the COVID-19 pandemic, they have been used before the pandemic to study influenza-associated deaths[8] and heat-related mortality,[9] and more recently to compare US mortality with the mortality of peer nations.[10,11] These applications are valuable because they convert abstract public health issues into a quantity that is easy to understand for researchers across different fields, policymakers, and the general public.

Despite its many strengths, excess mortality as a metric also has some weaknesses. Death is often preceded by visible symptoms and, in the case of a viral disease, by an infection, possibly resulting in hospitalization. As such, other metrics like test positivity, percentage of emergency department visits diagnosed as COVID-19, hospitalizations, and severe acute respiratory syndrome coronavirus 2 (SARS-CoV-2) RNA levels in wastewater provide better early indicators of the evolution of a health emergency. In addition, deaths are usually reported and made available to researchers with a lag. For example, mortality data for the United States are only 65% complete within two weeks and 85% after four weeks, and remain only 95% complete after eight weeks.[12] These reporting lags further limit the usefulness of excess mortality as a real-time indicator. However, most alternative indicators do not guarantee complete coverage and, aside from hospitalizations, are more useful in measuring the spread rather than in assessing the intensity of a health emergency. Excess mortality thus stands out as a tool to retrospectively evaluate the effectiveness of measures aimed at reducing the negative health impact of a health emergency.

The numerous advantages of the excess mortality metric suggest that it is likely to remain an essential tool for monitoring emerging threats to population health moving forward. Future research should continue to develop, refine, and standardize excess mortality modeling tools to assist with future public health preparedness and response efforts. AJPH

CORRESPONDENCE

Correspondence should be sent to Andrew C. Stokes, 801 Massachusetts Ave, Crosstown Building 362, Boston, MA 02118 (e-mail: acstokes@bu.edu). Reprints can be ordered at https://ajph.org by clicking the "Reprints" link.

PUBLICATION INFORMATION

Full Citation: Paglino E, Stokes AC. Excess mortality as a tool to monitor the evolution of health emergencies: choices, challenges, and future directions. *Am J Public Health*. 2024;114(6): 583–586.

Acceptance Date: March 7, 2024.

DOI: https://doi.org/10.2105/AJPH.2024.307661

ORCID iD:

Eugenio Paglino https://orcid.org/0000-0001-8733-6460

Andrew C. Stokes https://orcid.org/0000-0002-8502-3636

CONTRIBUTORS

E. Paglino and A. C. Stokes conceptualized, drafted, and revised the editorial.

ACKNOWLEDGMENTS

Support for this work came from grants received from Robert Wood Johnson Foundation (77521); the National Institutes of Health, National Institute on Aging (R01-AG060115-04S1); the W. K. Kellogg Foundation (P-6007864-2022); and the National Science Foundation (CCF-2200052).

We wish to thank Rafeya Raquib for her valuable contributions to the design of the visualization. We gratefully acknowledge the resources provided by the Center on Emerging Infectious Diseases at Boston University and the International Max Planck Research School for Population, Health, and Data Science.

Note. The interpretations, conclusions, and recommendations in this work are those of the authors and do not necessarily represent the views of the study sponsors.

CONFLICTS OF INTEREST

The authors have no conflicts of interest to report.

REFERENCES

1. Krieger N, Chen JT, Waterman PD. Excess mortality in men and women in Massachusetts during the COVID-19 pandemic. *Lancet.* 2020;395(10240):1829. https://doi.org/10.1016/S0140-6736(20)31234-4
2. Woolf SH, Chapman DA, Sabo RT, Zimmerman EB. Excess deaths from COVID-19 and other causes in the US, March 1, 2020, to January 2, 2021. *JAMA.* 2021;325(17):1786–1789. https://doi.org/10.1001/jama.2021.5199
3. Faust JS, Krumholz HM, Du C, et al. All-cause excess mortality and COVID-19–related mortality among US adults aged 25–44 years, March–July 2020. *JAMA.* 2021;325(8):785–787. https://doi.org/10.1001/jama.2020.24243
4. Konstantinoudis G, Cameletti M, Gómez-Rubio V, et al. Regional excess mortality during the 2020 COVID-19 pandemic in five European countries. *Nat Commun.* 2022;13(1):482. https://doi.org/10.1038/s41467-022-28157-3
5. Paglino E, Lundberg DJ, Zhou Z, et al. Monthly excess mortality across counties in the United States during the COVID-19 pandemic, March 2020 to February 2022. *Sci Adv.* 2023;9(25):eadf9742. https://doi.org/10.1126/sciadv.adf9742
6. Nepomuceno MR, Klimkin I, Jdanov DA, Alustiza-Galarza A, Shkolnikov VM. Sensitivity analysis of excess mortality due to the COVID-19 pandemic. *Popul Dev Rev.* 2022;48(2):279–302. https://doi.org/10.1111/padr.12475
7. Heuveline P, Tzen M. Beyond deaths per capita: comparative COVID-19 mortality indicators. *BMJ Open.* 2021;11(3):e042934. https://doi.org/10.1136/bmjopen-2020-042934
8. Thompson WW, Weintraub E, Dhankhar P, et al. Estimates of US influenza-associated deaths made using four different methods. *Influenza Other Respir Viruses.* 2009;3(1):37–49. https://doi.org/10.1111/j.1750-2659.2009.00073.x
9. Kosatsky T. The 2003 European heat waves. *Euro Surveill.* 2005;10(7):3–4. https://doi.org/10.2807/esm.10.07.00552-en
10. Preston SH, Vierboom YC. Excess mortality in the United States in the 21st century. *Proc Natl Acad Sci USA.* 2021;118(16):e2024850118. https://doi.org/10.1073/pnas.2024850118
11. Bor J, Stokes AC, Raifman J, et al. Missing Americans: early death in the United States—1933–2021. *PNAS Nexus.* 2023;2(6):gad173. https://doi.org/10.1093/pnasnexus/pgad173
12. Centers for Disease Control and Prevention. Technical notes. Provisional death counts for COVID-19. September 28, 2023. Available at: https://www.cdc.gov/nchs/nvss/vsrr/covid19/tech_notes.htm. Accessed January 28, 2024.

Local Impact From International Crises: Unregulated Drug Toxicity During the COVID-19 Pandemic in British Columbia, Canada

Samuel Tobias, MSc, Jane A. Buxton, MBBS, MHSc, and Lianping Ti, PhD

ABOUT THE AUTHORS

Samuel Tobias is with the School of Population and Public Health, University of British Columbia, and the British Columbia Centre on Substance Use, Vancouver, Canada. Jane A. Buxton is with the School of Population and Public Health, University of British Columbia. Lianping Ti is with the Department of Medicine, University of British Columbia, and the British Columbia Centre on Substance Use.

See also Excess Mortality Calculations: Methods and Uses, pp. 575–609.

The first few months of the COVID-19 pandemic brought uncertainty and instability for people around the world. Public health interventions primarily centered around physical distancing measures that disproportionately affected structurally vulnerable populations, including people who use drugs, exacerbated social isolation by disrupting established routines and networks. The article in this issue of *AJPH* by Chandra et al. (p. 599) is the first to describe the excess drug-related deaths attributable to the COVID-19 pandemic in the United States at a local (county-level) scale. We applaud the authors for bringing to light the geographic variability in excess drug-related mortality on a granular level.

Chandra et al. propose four main factors that "interacted and differentially affected" overdose mortality rates across the United States through the first 18 months of the COVID-19 pandemic: an overburdened health system, pandemic-related socio-behavioral factors, the growing availability of potent drugs, and pandemic period changes to supply and demand. We describe how each of these factors contributed to increased illicit drug–related mortality in British Columbia (BC), Canada.

AN OVERBURDENED HEALTH SYSTEM

In BC, "accidental overdose" is now referred to as "illicit drug toxicity," emphasizing the unpredictable nature of the unregulated drug supply and the systemic forces that contribute to drug-related risk. The term "accidental" connotes a level of chance, which is incongruous because these deaths are preventable. Between 2013 and 2018, the rise in illicit drug toxicity was primarily driven by the proliferation of illicitly manufactured fentanyl. A turning point was marked in 2019 as the province began to exhibit signs of amelioration. Illicit drug–related mortality rates fell through 2019,[1] attributed to public health responses such as the expansion of the provincial take-home naloxone program and the introduction of provincially exempted overdose prevention sites for supervised drug consumption.[2] A key aspect of the provincial response has been peer-led interventions; however, peers (individuals with lived or living experience of substance use), who are at increased risk of burnout, reached critical levels of compassion fatigue during the pandemic.[3]

Following the declaration of the COVID-19 public health emergency in BC, deaths caused by illicit drug toxicity more than doubled compared with the immediate prepandemic months, and in the years since have remained at all-time highs.[1] This strain has been borne largely by peer responders on the front lines of the crisis. Peers are well equipped to respond to the drug poisoning crisis, yet are not appropriately supported by the greater system. There exists a lack of recognition, emotional support, and adequate pay.[3]

SOCIAL ISOLATION

Physical distancing measures led to increased solitary drug use, a significant risk factor for illicit drug–related mortality. This concern was the motivating factor for the release of the province's unique risk mitigation guidance for prescribers, which strongly recommended expanded access (through longer-term prescriptions and home deliveries) of prescribed pharmaceutical alternatives to the unregulated drug supply for those at the highest risks of both

AJPH June 2024, Vol. 114, No. 6

COVID-19 infection and illicit drug toxicity.[4] Although a recent study found a protective effect of these opioid prescriptions on mortality outcomes,[4] low rates of access among people with opioid use disorder in the province (7.6%) may have resulted in little impact to overall mortality at the population level. In addition, pandemic-related distancing mandates led to a dramatic drop in visits to harm reduction sites and decreased access to supervised consumption services (57% reduction from January to April 2020).[5] Given the known impact these supervised consumption sites have on preventing drug poisoning deaths,[2] the response to one public health emergency may have overshadowed another.

Indeed, over the first two years of the pandemic, illicit drug–related mortality surpassed COVID-19 deaths in BC. Although physical distancing measures surely played some role in increased acute drug-related risk, following the relaxation of these measures, drug-related mortality in BC has remained high—and even increased.[1] As such, other factors were likely more consequential. An analysis of demographics of those dying from illicit drug toxicity after the onset of the pandemic in BC highlighted how older individuals were most affected[6]; the authors pointed to obstacles faced by older people who use drugs in accessing essential medical services through pandemic-related disruptions, including isolation felt from adhering to physical distancing orders.

A CHANGING DRUG SUPPLY

BC's unregulated drug supply started evolving prior to the COVID-19 pandemic, but these changes have certainly been accelerated by it. Fentanyl has been the predominant opioid in BC's unregulated opioid supply since at least 2016, when fentanyl was found in 67% of postmortem toxicology tests conducted on illicit drug toxicity decedents.[1] The fentanyl supply was shown to be consistent and correlated over time prior to the pandemic, but an interrupted time-series analysis of community drug-checking samples in Vancouver, BC showed that the onset of the COVID-19 pandemic was associated with increased variability, and therefore unpredictability, of fentanyl concentrations in available drugs.[7] Over this same time period, unregulated opioids were increasingly adulterated with potent, novel benzodiazepines such as etizolam, flubromazolam, and flualprazolam across the province. In fact, after the percentage of decedents with novel benzodiazepines in their postmortem toxicology increased steadily in 2020, it reached more than 50% in some months in early 2021.[8] The presence of these benzodiazepines in polysubstance mixtures with opioids increases the risk of overdose and, concerningly, can lead to periods of prolonged sedation and difficulty rousing individuals exposed. Their presence in the unregulated drug supply remains a continued concern. Of additional note, a recent analysis from BC identified a significant, positive relationship between circulating fentanyl concentrations in the drug supply and illicit drug–related mortality in the same setting.[9] Although by no means can the fentanyl supply be considered reliable, as it is impossible to know the concentration of a batch when purchased from the unregulated market, concentrations at an aggregate have shown consistent patterns. Supply shocks, like the one caused by the intersecting influences associated with the pandemic, disrupted this consistency, putting people at heightened risk for exposure to unexpectedly high concentrations of fentanyl.[7]

SUPPLY DISRUPTIONS

The causal link between COVID-19 and changes to the drug supply has not yet been established in BC. Although Chandra et al. propose border closures and disruptions, data from the Canada Border Services Agency show how fentanyl seizures were already declining prior to COVID-19 and that fentanyl is increasingly produced domestically.[10,11] Smaller-scale drug preparation (i.e., the settings where drugs are weighed and packaged for distribution) were likely affected by physical distancing orders, in turn leading to downstream supply changes. Benzodiazepine adulteration of opioids, which likely started as a supply side approach to enhance depressive effects and augment the need for fentanyl, has become desired by some and is now driven by demand.

CONCLUSION

Illicit drug–related mortality occurs at the confluence of many variable factors. We agree with Chandra et al. that local responses are needed as the effects of this crisis are borne too heavily by some communities. To prevent death, proactive monitoring of local mortality trends is essential, but equally imperative is broadening our scope beyond mere death statistics. By incorporating comprehensive administrative data and monitoring changes to the unregulated drug supply, resources can be allocated effectively to communities in need. By understanding the nuances of the ongoing crisis at the local level, we can implement preventive and harm-reducing measures that address the root causes of illicit drug toxicity. AJPH

CORRESPONDENCE

Correspondence should be sent to Samuel Tobias, 400–1045 Howe St., Vancouver, British Columbia, Canada (e-mail: samuel.tobias@bccsu.ubc.ca). Reprints can be ordered at http://www.ajph.org by clicking the "Reprints" link.

PUBLICATION INFORMATION

Full Citation: Tobias S, Buxton JA, Ti L. Local impact from international crises: unregulated drug toxicity during the COVID-19 pandemic in British Columbia, Canada. *Am J Public Health*. 2024;114(6):587–589.

Acceptance Date: March 25, 2024.

DOI: https://doi.org/10.2105/AJPH.2024.307673

ORCID iD:
Samuel Tobias https://orcid.org/0000-0001-6051-8950

CONTRIBUTORS

S. Tobias conceptualized the article and prepared the first draft. J. A. Buxton and L. Ti provided critical feedback and approved the final version.

ACKNOWLEDGMENTS

S. Tobias is supported by a Four Year Doctoral Fellowship from the University of British Columbia.

CONFLICTS OF INTEREST

The authors have no conflicts of interest to declare.

REFERENCES

1. British Columbia Coroners Service. Illicit drug toxicity deaths in British Columbia. January 24, 2024. Available at: https://www2.gov.bc.ca/gov/content/life-events/death/coroners-service/statistical-reports. Accessed February 7, 2024.
2. Irvine MA, Kuo M, Buxton JA, et al. Modelling the combined impact of interventions in averting deaths during a synthetic-opioid overdose epidemic. *Addiction*. 2019;114(9):1602–1613. https://doi.org/10.1111/add.14664
3. Mamdani Z, Loyal JP, Xavier J, et al. "We are the first responders": overdose response experiences and perspectives among peers in British Columbia. *Drugs Educ Prev Policy*. 2024;31(1):91–104. https://doi.org/10.1080/09687637.2022.2132134
4. Slaunwhite A, Min JE, Palis H, et al. Effect of Risk Mitigation Guidance for opioid and stimulant dispensations on mortality and acute care visits during dual public health emergencies: retrospective cohort study. *BMJ*. 2024;384:e076336. https://doi.org/10.1136/bmj-2023-076336
5. British Columbia Centre for Disease Control. Unregulated Drug Poisoning Emergency Dashboard. January 12, 2024. Available at: http://www.bccdc.ca/health-professionals/data-reports/substance-use-harm-reduction-dashboard. Accessed February 7, 2024.
6. Palis H, Bélair MA, Hu K, Tu A, Buxton J, Slaunwhite A. Overdose deaths and the COVID-19 pandemic in British Columbia, Canada. *Drug Alcohol Rev*. 2022;41(4):912–917. https://doi.org/10.1111/dar.13424
7. Tobias S, Grant CJ, Laing R, et al. What impact did the COVID-19 pandemic have on the variability of fentanyl concentrations in the Vancouver, Canada illicit drug supply? An interrupted time-series analysis. *BMJ Public Health*. 2023;1(1):e000197. https://doi.org/10.1136/bmjph-2023-000197
8. British Columbia Coroners Service. Illicit drug toxicity type of drug data (to December 31, 2022). Ministry of Public Safety and Solicitor General. 2023. Available at: https://www2.gov.bc.ca/assets/gov/birth-adoption-death-marriage-and-divorce/deaths/coroners-service/statistical/illicit-drug-type.pdf. Accessed February 17, 2024.
9. Kennedy MC, Dong H, Tobias S, et al. Fentanyl concentration in drug checking samples and risk of overdose death in Vancouver, Canada. *Am J Prev Med*. 2024;66(1):10–17. https://doi.org/10.1016/j.amepre.2023.08.016
10. Government of Canada. Canada Border Services Agency seizures. February 15, 2024. Available at: https://www.cbsa-asfc.gc.ca/security-securite/seizure-saisie-eng.html. Accessed February 17, 2024.
11. Ovalle D, Miroff N. Fentanyl super labs in Canada pose new threat for US opioid epidemic. *Washington Post*. December 24, 2023. Available at: https://www.washingtonpost.com/health/2023/12/24/fentanyl-labs-canada-threat-to-us/#. Accessed February 6, 2024.

Overdose and COVID-19 in Baja California, Mexico: The Need for New Methodologies for Understanding Local Trends

Jaime Arredondo Sanchez Lira, PhD, MA, and David Goodman-Meza, MD, MAS

ABOUT THE AUTHORS

Jaime Arredondo Sanchez Lira is an assistant professor at the School of Public Health and Social Policy, University of Victoria, British Columbia, Canada, and a Canada research chair on substance use and health systems at the Canadian Institute of Substance Use Research. David Goodman-Meza is with the Department of Medicine, David Geffen School of Medicine at University of California, Los Angeles.

See also Excess Mortality Calculations: Methods and Uses, pp. 575–609.

AJPH June 2024, Vol. 114, No. 6

Throughout North America, the illicit drug supply's shift to illicitly manufactured fentanyl (IMF) has fueled a multiwave overdose crisis.[1] In response to the public health crisis, several jurisdictions in the United States and Canada adopted a range of harm reduction strategies. These strategies include take-home naloxone programs, community drug checking services, increased access to medications for opioid use disorder, and the prescription of safe supply medications.

In Mexico, the implementation of harm reduction interventions has been extremely limited.[2] Faced with opposition at various government levels, local harm reduction programs have struggled to emerge or operate at full scale. Meanwhile, certain Mexican border areas are experiencing a rapid emergence of IMF in their local drug supply,[3] leading to a spike in overdoses and an increase in other negative health outcomes for people who use drugs.

AN UNKNOWN CRISIS

The Mexican border cities of Tijuana and Mexicali, both neighboring California, have historically been a major route for drug trafficking of heroin, cocaine, and methamphetamines, with local drug consumption patterns influenced by their geographic proximity to the United States.[4] In the last few years, these cities have also seen higher levels of overdose cases according to limited data from local harm reduction organizations,[5] despite the lack of overdoses reported in official Mexican government statistics. However, according to official sources, in all of Mexico, in 2019, only 11 deaths were related to opioids, eight to cocaine, 13 to other stimulants (e.g., methamphetamine), and 167 to polysubstance use.[6] For a country of more than 120 million people where substance use is known, these numbers are surprisingly low, in spite of the increases in the Baja California cities.

Few studies in Mexico have attempted to estimate the magnitude of overdoses in the country, with only a handful focused on this phenomenon during the COVID-19 pandemic. In 2022, a study by Magis Rodríguez et al. combined overdose reporting by community organizations, news reports, emergency services statistics, and numbers from the federal government's System of Epidemiological Surveillance of Addictions to estimate fatal and nonfatal overdoses in the country between 2019 and 2020. The research team estimated that there were more than 20 000 nonfatal overdoses and proposed two mortality scenarios—low and high—with rates ranging from 0.6% to 5%, depending on the parameters used.[7]

Our previous research at the community level, using case report forms collected between 2019 and 2021 in the context of an overdose reversal program in the city of Mexicali, documented a 30% increase in reported overdoses following the declaration of a public health emergency because of COVID-19.[5] This situation coincided with an increase of IMF in the local drug supply, as indicated by the drug testing program set up by the local harm reduction organization.[8] These numbers in overdose and fentanyl detection[9] have not been seen in other Mexican cities and emphasize the need to focus on local information to understand the heterogeneity of overdoses in different regions, as suggested by Chandra et al. in this issue of *AJPH* (p. 599), in the United States.

During the early stages of the public health emergency, we conducted research in collaboration with community organizations that provide services to vulnerable populations in the city of Tijuana. This was done alongside other academic partners from the National University in Mexico City and the

University of California, San Diego. Our goal was to understand the prevalence and correlates of COVID-19 among female sex workers to develop better strategies for preventing infection. Although seroprevalence among the general population in the city indicated a prevalence of 22%, our small pilot sample revealed a rate nearly twice as high. This finding underscores the greater burden of the disease on this highly stigmatized and vulnerable population, a trend that could also be expected for other groups such as people who use drugs. Many areas in the country lack the community-based organizations and academic resources necessary to conduct local studies assessing the pandemic's impact on their cities.

A PATH FORWARD

The use of cause-specific death data to understand overdoses in the United States has produced research that allows for an understanding of regional dynamics. For example, a county-level study by Palau et al.[10] shows how the overdose epidemic has progressed on the northern side of the US–Mexico border, linking it to specific socioeconomic variables that can help recognize the structural determinants of the problem. However, the modeling of the excess fatal overdoses using CDC WONDER data by substance and geography provides a methodological path for understanding the granular differences that we might have missed from other analyses.

To understand the excess mortality attributable to COVID-19 in Mexico, a group of researchers used cause-specific death data, estimating almost 600 000 lives lost in excess.[11] Although the team in Mexico did not include substance use as a specific cause group, the current research by Chandra et al. could serve as an example to be applied to the Mexican context. This additional research of excess of mortality attributable to overdose using death certificates could help emphasize the need to develop a decentralized overdose prevention strategy that recognizes the geographical differences when dealing with the negative consequences of substance use.[12]

As we attempt to understand the impact of COVID-19 on our communities, particularly its influence on the risk of overdoses in North America, it is essential to recognize the value of using similar methodological tools that can provide insights on a local scale. For instance, it is important to ensure that forensic medical services are trained and equipped with the necessary tools to thoroughly investigate all suspected overdose cases, using consistent methods across borders. Community-based organizations play a crucial role in preventing fatal overdoses; thus, standardizing forms for naloxone use can help in understanding variations not only at the county level but also within cities in terms of geographic and substance type trends. Finally, enhancing collaboration among research institutions, public health offices, and harm reduction service organizations from Mexico, Canada, and the United States is crucial for developing unified responses and facilitating the sharing of best practices. AJPH

CORRESPONDENCE

Correspondence should be sent to Jaime Arredondo Sanchez Lira, Canadian Institute for Substance Use Research (CISUR), 2300 McKenzie Ave, Victoria, BC V8N 5M8, Canada (e-mail: jaimeasl@uvic.ca). Reprints can be ordered at https://ajph.org by clicking the "Reprints" link.

PUBLICATION INFORMATION

Full Citation: Arredondo Sanchez Lira J, Goodman-Meza D. Overdose and COVID-19 in Baja California, Mexico: the need for new methodologies for understanding local trends. *Am J Public Health*. 2024;114(6): 590–592.

Acceptance Date: March 25, 2024.

DOI: https://doi.org/10.2105/AJPH.2024.307672

CONTRIBUTORS

Both authors contributed equally to this editorial.

ACKNOWLEDGMENTS

This research was undertaken, in part, thanks to funding from the Canada Research Chairs Program. D. Goodman-Meza was supported by the US National Institute on Drug Abuse (grant K08 DA048163, PI: Goodman-Meza) and by the US National Institute on Mental Health (grant P30 MH58107, PI: Shoptaw).

We extend our gratitude to the harm reduction organizations offering overdose prevention services across the country, especially to the dedicated teams at Verter AC in Mexicali and Prevencasa AC in Tijuana. Their life-saving efforts are a reminder of the ongoing challenges faced by civil society in Mexico and the significant risks drug users face in the nation.

CONFLICTS OF INTEREST

The authors declare no conflicts of interest.

REFERENCES

1. Ciccarone D. The rise of illicit fentanyls, stimulants and the fourth wave of the opioid overdose crisis. *Curr Opin Psychiatry*. 2021;34(4):344–350. https://doi.org/10.1097/YCO.0000000000000717
2. Beletsky L, Baker P, Arredondo J, et al. The global health and equity imperative for safe consumption facilities. *Lancet*. 2018;392(10147):553–554. https://doi.org/10.1016/S0140-6736(18)31469-7
3. Friedman J, Bourgois P, Godvin M, et al. The introduction of fentanyl on the US–Mexico border: an ethnographic account triangulated with drug checking data from Tijuana. *Int J Drug Policy*. 2022;104: 103678. https://doi.org/10.1016/j.drugpo.2022.103678
4. Bucardo J, Brouwer KC, Magis-Rodríguez C, et al. Historical trends in the production and consumption of illicit drugs in Mexico: implications for the prevention of blood borne infections. *Drug Alcohol Depend*. 2005;79(3):281–293. https://doi.org/10.1016/j.drugalcdep.2005.02.003
5. Goodman-Meza D, Slim S, Angulo L, et al. Impact of an overdose reversal program in the context of a safe consumption site in Northern Mexico [erratum in *Drug Alcohol Depend Rep*. 2022;4: 100079]. *Drug Alcohol Depend Rep*. 2021;2:100021. https://doi.org/10.1016/j.dadr.2021.100021
6. CONADIC. Report on the situation of mental health and the consumption of psychoactive substances in Mexico [in Spanish]. 2021.

Available at: https://www.gob.mx/cms/uploads/attachment/file/648021/INFORME_PAIS_2021.pdf. Accessed March 10, 2024.

7. Magis Rodríguez CL, García A, Meza Hernández JA, et al. Fatal and non-fatal overdoses due to opioid consumption in the context of the COVID-19 pandemic in northern Mexico [in Spanish]. *Revista UNAM: Boletín sobre COVID-19.* 2022;3(28).
8. Goodman-Meza D, Arredondo J, Slim S, et al. Behavior change after fentanyl testing at a safe consumption space for women in Northern Mexico: a pilot study. *Int J Drug Policy.* 2022;106:103745. https://doi.org/10.1016/j.drugpo.2022.103745
9. Arredondo J, Garcia de Loera A, Garcia de Loera L, Gonzalez P, Chavez A, Zwitser G. Testing stimulants: detection of fentanyl and harm reduction in four cities in Mexico [in Spanish]. Programa de Política de Drogas. 2022. Available at: https://politicadedrogas.org/site/proyecto/id/26.html. Accessed March 10, 2024.
10. Palau CB, Akikuni M, Latsky-Campbell B, Wagner J. The drug overdose epidemic in the US–Mexico border region: shifts, progression, and community characteristics. *Subst Use Misuse.* 2024;59(2):184–192. https://doi.org/10.1080/10826084.2023.2267110
11. Palacio-Mejía LS, Hernández-Ávila JE, Hernández-Ávila M, et al. Leading causes of excess mortality in Mexico during the COVID-19 pandemic 2020-2021: a death certificates study in a middle-income country. *Lancet Reg Health Am.* 2022;13:100303. https://doi.org/10.1016/j.lana.2022.100303
12. Bejarano Romero R, Arredondo Sánchez-Lira J, Slim Pasaran S, et al. Implementing a decentralized opioid overdose prevention strategy in Mexico, a pending public policy issue. *Lancet Reg Health Am.* 2023;23:100535. https://doi.org/10.1016/j.lana.2023.100535

Excess Mortality Calculations to Assess the Impact of the COVID-19 Pandemic: Concepts and Methodological Issues

Jan P. Vandenbroucke, MD, PhD, and Neil Pearce, PhD

See also Excess Mortality Calculations: Methods and Uses, pp. 575–609.

We discuss some intriguing methodological aspects of excess mortality analyses, which have been widely used to describe the impact of the COVID-19 pandemic. We describe the main ways of presenting excess mortality: as a mortality rate (incidence rate) or as a percentage increase (relative risk or rate ratio).

We discuss what should be regarded as the null value of excess mortality (i.e., when countries or regions can be judged as having fared equally well) and when age and sex standardization, adjustment for other determinants of the spread of a pandemic, or both is necessary. We discuss the level of detail by time and place and person that may be necessary. We note that an excess mortality comparison is essentially a difference-in-differences analysis.

We conclude that, although one cannot rule out using excess mortality analyses for causal effect estimates, such analyses will remain most fruitful for generating hypotheses about both the efficiency of measures to curtail the pandemic and factors that cannot be influenced. Nevertheless, a judicious use of arguments and counterarguments can then lead to identifying best practices for various situations.
(*Am J Public Health*. 2024;114(6):593–598. https://doi.org/10.2105/AJPH.2024.307572)

AJPH June 2024, Vol. 114, No. 6

Excess mortality analyses have been widely used with regard to the COVID-19 pandemic, apparently to compare how different countries fared. For example, according to the calculations by Islam et al.,[1] Norway, Denmark, and New Zealand have shown negative excess mortality during the pandemic (i.e., mortality was lower than expected on the basis of the prepandemic mortality rates). As a corollary, life expectancy increased during the pandemic in Norway, South Korea, Taiwan, and New Zealand, with New Zealand showing a remarkable 0.5 years of increase in life expectancy during the single year 2020.[2] All other countries with comparable data experienced excess mortality and decreases in life expectancy, some very large: both Russia and the United States showed decreases in life expectancy of more than 2 life-years.[2]

The measure of excess total mortality is least susceptible to some of the potential biases of other measures of the COVID-19 pandemic's impact.[3] It is not susceptible to the vagaries of being tested, of being diagnosed, or of cause-of-death classifications. There are major international differences and differences over time in countries in how death from COVID-19 is defined, identified, and recorded, making international comparisons and time trend comparisons difficult and questionable.

By contrast, total mortality is relatively easy to identify and report, and excess mortality is also relatively easy to calculate (e.g., by comparing total mortality during the pandemic with that expected on the basis of mortality rates during prepandemic years). Thus, it can be argued that excess mortality is the definitive measure of the net effects of the pandemic and the policy measures adopted to mitigate it. Therefore, it is deeply interesting and informative to make comparisons between countries, regions, and age groups and other subgroups using measures of excess mortality. However, the apparent simplicity of excess mortality analyses hides complexities in thinking about how to present and compare excess mortality (e.g., between different times, different places, or different types of people).

The clear negative excess mortality in countries such as New Zealand, Norway, and Taiwan is intriguing and perhaps provides the benchmark against which other countries should be compared. However, it also illustrates the difficulties of interpreting excess mortality estimates from a single country. The example of New Zealand is illustrative. Clearly, the antipandemic measures adopted in New Zealand resulted in reductions in total mortality. These measures included quarantine at the borders that was implemented for more than 2 years coupled with temporary lockdowns and social distancing. These latter measures appear to have been less severe and less prolonged in New Zealand than in most European and North American countries. This is because an initial period of lockdown and social distancing initially eliminated the virus—for a long period, the few cases of COVID-19 were imported and arose among those quarantined or staff working in quarantine and their close contacts—and the few outbreaks were quickly managed.

In fact, New Zealand experienced negative excess mortality both during the short lockdown period (of about 2 months) and during the subsequent periods when there were few restrictions besides quarantine at the border. The reasons for this likely include reductions in mortality from other causes, as there were very few deaths from COVID-19 in New Zealand before the advent of the omicron strain. Analogously, it is known that early in an economic depression, total mortality decreases; the reasons for this are not clear but may include reductions in deaths from accidents, cardiovascular disease, and alcohol-related diseases.[4] In addition, because of the COVID-19 prevention measures, there may have been less mortality from winter influenza, owing to less transmission of infections in general, and from suicide.[5]

According to New Zealand researchers, there was a complete absence of a winter peak in mortality in the year 2020 (extended winter in New Zealand being the months May–October). Their analyses also made it possible to ascribe the absence of a winter peak in mortality to the measures taken to prohibit the spread of viral respiratory infections in general and not to warmer winters.[6] Moreover, these researchers indicate the major public health importance of respiratory infections in causing a winter peak of total mortality, which may translate to several different causes of death (e.g., in persons with long-standing cardiovascular or respiratory diseases whose final illness is triggered by a respiratory infection).

By contrast, countries that undertook pandemic measures later or with less vigor would be expected to have a larger number of COVID-19 deaths, even if these deaths were offset by reduced mortality from other infectious or other causes attributable to antipandemic measures.[7] It is, therefore, tempting to also examine cause-specific excess deaths in hopes of identifying excess COVID-19–specific deaths and fewer (or more) deaths from other causes. However, the results of such calculations and comparisons are questionable because of potential misclassification of deaths from other causes (e.g., respiratory disease, heart disease) as COVID-19 deaths and vice versa.

Furthermore, the practice of coding cause-specific deaths during the pandemic (i.e., the attribution of death to COVID-19 in, e.g., older people with chronic heart or lung conditions) is likely to have varied between countries. Conversely, disruption of medical services when hospitals were overwhelmed with COVID-19 patients may have caused deaths from other diseases because of delayed care, particularly in countries where the pandemic raged.[8–11] Therefore, examination of cause-specific excess mortality, although of interest, may not provide definitive findings, particularly when comparing countries.

Thus, direct international comparisons and time trend comparisons of COVID-19 death rates are questionable because of differences in identifying and coding COVID-19 deaths across countries and periods.[3] An excess mortality approach has some obvious advantages but may also be misleading if an excess of COVID-19 deaths is masked by a decrease (perhaps real, perhaps only apparent because of shifts in coding) of deaths from other causes. Furthermore, there is no placebo reference category (i.e., a country that adopted no COVID-19 measures at all), at least not in high-income countries.

A DIFFERENCE-IN-DIFFERENCES APPROACH

A comparison of excess mortality rates between countries and between population subgroups (e.g., socioeconomic level) amounts to a difference-in-differences (DiD) analysis in which 2 or more countries are compared with regard to their changes in total mortality as a result of the pandemic and the policy responses to it. This approach can also be used for other health outcomes. For example, a DiD approach has recently been used to assess the effects of lifting universal masking in schools on severe acute respiratory syndrome coronavirus 2 (SARS-CoV-2) infection rates.[12] The authors assessed the effects of masking policy changes, rather than directly estimating the effects of masking itself.

Although a formal DiD analysis seems to be a newer tool used in epidemiology, it is not a new method, as it may come naturally when investigating the course of diseases in populations. The more formalized way of dealing with DiD analyses has been widely used in econometrics. According to present-day views, DiD analyses in epidemiology permit us to obtain valid answers when there is potentially considerable unmeasured or unmeasurable confounding.[13] They compare the mean change in outcome (in this case, national death rates) over time between populations; usually they are termed "exposed" and "unexposed," but in the current context one is simply comparing different sets of COVID-19 policies. The populations may be countries or parts of countries, or they may be limited to certain age categories, sex categories, or both.

The underlying assumption of such analyses is that baseline (i.e., prepandemic) differences in outcome (i.e., death rates) reflect differences in various population-level risk factors (acting as confounders and effect modifiers) and that rates of change in death rates are similar in the countries that are compared until the arrival of the pandemic, or at least that any future changes are predictable (e.g., if a country has decreasing prepandemic mortality, this can be considered in the estimation of predicted mortality for the pandemic period). In a World Bank review, this was formulated by saying, "The validity of the difference-in-differences approach relies on the equal trends assumption, or rather the assumption that no time-varying differences exist between the treatment and control groups."[14] Under this assumption, the DiD between observed and expected mortality (based on prepandemic levels and time trends) during the pandemic period reflects the effects of different COVID-19 mitigation policies in different societies.

CALCULATION OF EXCESS TOTAL MORTALITY

A further issue is how excess mortality is defined and measured. An excess can be estimated in absolute numbers (total number of excess deaths), as an excess mortality rate, or as a relative excess (e.g., the excess mortality as a percentage of the expected mortality). In the Appendix (available as a supplement to the online version of this article at http://www.ajph.org), we describe calculations of excess mortality rates and relative excess (and variants thereof). However, we wish to focus here on the different uses of a rate difference type of calculation versus a relative risk (RR) type of calculation (i.e., the excess mortality rate vs the relative excess). In some situations, the total crude numbers of events may also be of interest.

In general, considerations about the choice between a rate difference measure (e.g., excess mortality rate) and a rate ratio measure (e.g., relative excess, RR, percentages) are similar to the considerations for using these measures more generally in epidemiology and public health. Both have advantages and disadvantages. In general, changes in rates (and risks) give a better picture of the total burden of disease and may therefore be the best for public health evaluation, whereas relative changes may be of more interest in terms of causal inference.[15] Moreover, there is value in presenting absolute numbers: a relative excess deaths measure, or even a rate difference, may undermine the realization of a vast loss of human lives. For example, 5% excess death may seem like "not too much," but it may translate to a large number at the whole-population level. Therefore, it seems like good practice to always show absolute numbers even when researchers estimated excess deaths on a RR or rate scale.

Although the focus is usually on total mortality, in part to avoid problems of cause-of-death classification, estimation of excess mortality in terms of incidence rates could also be used for individual causes of death in a country. For COVID-19 deaths, for which the incidence rate before December 2019 was zero, the difference in mortality rates amounts to registered COVID-19 mortality. For each country (or region, etc.) such a calculation has the advantage that increases or decreases of each cause of death can be mutually compared in that country. This permits insight into what happened to cause of death certification in a particular country during the COVID-19 pandemic. For example, cause-specific mortality is not yet available for New Zealand for the pandemic period, but it will be useful to eventually examine which causes of death (in addition to winter influenza and other winter infections) contributed to the overall negative excess mortality.

For a single comparison, over time or between just 2 countries or groups of people, it may not matter greatly whether a ratio or a difference in incidence rates is chosen to express excess mortality. However, when multiple countries are compared, an excess mortality rate analysis is likely to be the most informative.[1] Excess mortality in terms of mortality rates is related to the calculation of changes in life expectancy, which is perhaps the ultimate comparison of the COVID-19 pandemic's impact.[2] As is generally known from discussions of RRs versus absolute risks, depending on the height of the baseline risk (i.e., the mortality in prepandemic years), the picture given by an array of RRs can be different from that of an array of absolute risks (see the Appendix for an example).

NULL VALUE OF EXCESS MORTALITY

Even in the simplest situation (i.e., comparing 2 countries), what exactly constitutes the null value for excess mortality is debatable (i.e., how do we know that 2 countries did equally well?). Imagine 2 countries with very different prepandemic total mortality rates. Say there were 1000 deaths per million versus 2000 deaths per million, which has been the case for a decade or more. Both countries experienced the COVID-19 pandemic, and both took preventive measures. Suppose that the country with the lower mortality had an excess mortality rate of 50 per million. What should lead us to say that the other country did equally well? On an absolute scale, this would be true if it also had excess mortality of 50; on a proportional scale, this would be the case if it had excess mortality of 100. If the 2 countries had different prepandemic mortality rates, we can only be certain that they did equally well during the pandemic if both have zero excess mortality. This issue would become even more complicated if during the previous years the total mortality rates in both had been moving with increasing or decreasing slope.

By way of clinical analogy, comparing countries with very different baseline mortality rates is tantamount to comparing the effects of a treatment between patients with different prognoses, for example, antihypertensive treatment in patients with severe hypertension versus people with mild hypertension—the outcome being cerebrovascular accidents (CVA). Persons with severe hypertension will intrinsically have higher CVA rates, regardless of almost any treatment given. If their CVA rate was reduced to the rate of the treated patients with mild hypertension, that would be a tremendous accomplishment. Such an effect is likely to need far more aggressive therapy in patients with severe hypertension. Nevertheless, such a comparison is implied in some publications on international excess mortality, in which, for example, the United States figures together with Norway; however, these 2 countries have had different life expectancies from long before the pandemic.

A basic issue is whether the pandemic is thought to have added to or multiplied prepandemic death rates; in general, one would expect it to have added to death rates, and therefore excess rate is key (in both epidemiological and public health terms). However, we know from empirical data that COVID-19 death rates appear to be proportional to prepandemic death rates by age and sex and that death rates effectively doubled early in the pandemic; that is, if you caught COVID-19, your risk of death over the next month would have been about the same as your annual risk of death for your age group and sex.[16] Thus, it may be that one expects deaths to multiply, and therefore the excess rate ratio is key. By that reasoning, the safe conclusion may be that, when comparing 2 countries' excess mortality, we will find that 1 country had a worse mortality experience than the other, if it had a higher ratio increase than the other country did.

STANDARDIZING AND ADJUSTING

When comparing the efficacy of countries' pandemic protocols, whether the countries differ in age and sex composition should be considered, as should these variables' potential effect modification. One approach to tackling this problem is age or age–sex standardization. An example of an often used type of age standardization is the European Standard Population of 2013, a population the World Health Organization standardized for statistical purposes.[17] If there is effect modification by age or sex, it may be necessary to standardize for age, sex, or both to make valid comparisons between countries. However, if different measures were taken in countries with different age structures (e.g., a country with an older population adopted measures tailored to the elderly, whereas a country with a younger population adopted measures tailored to younger persons) then it may be inappropriate to standardize for age. In fact, the countries could be doing equally well in terms of adopting policies that were optimal for their own population, and an age-standardized analysis may indicate that 1 country is doing better than the other depending on whether the standardization gave more weight to the younger or older groups.

For other types of data interpretation, standardization may not be warranted, for example, when we want to determine if the patterns of change between 2 countries are similar or dissimilar. For instance, both the United States and the United Kingdom demonstrated increased mortality from causes other than COVID-19 during the pandemic.[8–11] This is apparently not the case in countries that were better at curtailing the pandemic. When describing such a difference of changes in mortality patterns, age standardization is moot.

Countries may also have different inherent risks for spreading SARS-CoV-2, such as population density, number of large households, and crowded living circumstances. This brings us back to the question of whether the pandemic would have affected different countries the same way in the absence of mitigation measures. The fact that huge differences in risk may exist even within a country is exemplified by a comparison between US states with high versus low vaccination rates or a comparison of the United States with European countries. Apparently, differences in socioeconomic or political circumstances can affect how the pandemic spreads.[18,19] This behooves us to contemplate controlling statistically for all such factors.

DETAILS AND TYPES OF CONTRASTS

Our discussion thus far has focused on comparisons between countries of annual excess mortality. However, early in the pandemic, excess mortality was also studied on a monthly and weekly basis to closely follow the evolution of the pandemic. The effectiveness of disease prevention and spread safeguards was most often evaluated in terms of weeks or months. Different time units may serve different purposes. Looking separately at 2020, when only public health measures were possible, and 2021, when vaccines became available, seems like a valuable subdivision. One recent review, however, lumped 2020 with 2021 and cast doubt on the different models used for calculation.[20] Such a combination hides, for example, Sweden's very high mortality in 2020, which was offset by a much lower mortality in 2021 (presumably because of increased mortality in particularly frail persons in the first year); this dramatic difference was not seen in other Nordic countries.

Analyses of parts of countries have also proven valuable; in Mexico, for example, regional socioeconomic inequalities led to differences in excess mortality,[21] as did racial/ethnic and age differences in the United States.[9] There have been insightful analyses of excess mortality among different occupations in the United Kingdom,[22] among adherents of different political parties in the United States,[19] and between men and women of all ages, men generally having higher mortalities.

CONCLUSIONS

Several aspects of excess mortality calculations and their comparison between countries or groups of people remain intriguing. These include the problem of the null value (when will we find that 2 countries did equally well?) and the issue of whether we should standardize or stratify for other factors that influence the spread, or the consequences, of a respiratory pandemic in different countries. What determined the decisions about which measures to take and what determined their successful implementation included such things as health conditions affected by socioeconomic circumstances and social inequalities, state structures, and governments and—within those—even political parties. Thus, in the end excess mortality comparisons will mostly serve descriptive epidemiologic purposes.[23] Nevertheless, such analyses may provide the best available evidence to estimate effects of government policies, as in the example of the DiD analysis of the lifting of masking requirements.[12]

As with any other analysis of observational data, any such estimates will rely on a number of assumptions, including that the expected mortality estimates are valid (taking into account previous mortality rates and their time trends) and that DiD between observed and expected mortality in 2 or more populations are being assessed on the appropriate (relative or absolute) scale and in the appropriate population groups or subgroups.

Thus, although one cannot rule out using such analyses for causal estimates about policies, they will perhaps remain most fruitful for generating hypotheses about the efficiency of measures to curtail the pandemic and about factors that cannot be influenced. A judicious use of arguments and counterarguments based on the existing knowledge of the spread of particular pandemic pathogens can then help us single out best practices for diverse situations. AJPH

ABOUT THE AUTHORS

Jan P. Vandenbroucke and Neil Pearce are with the Department of Medical Statistics, London School of Hygiene and Tropical Medicine, London, UK. Jan P. Vandenbroucke is also with the Department of Clinical Epidemiology, Aarhus University, Aarhus, Denmark, and the Department of Clinical Epidemiology, Leiden University Medical Center, Netherlands.

CORRESPONDENCE

Correspondence should be sent to Jan P. Vandenbroucke, Leiden University Medical Center, Department of Clinical Epidemiology, PO Box 9600, 2300 RC Leiden, The Netherlands (e-mail: J.P.Vandenbroucke@lumc.nl). Reprints can be ordered at http://www.ajph.org by clicking the "Reprints" link.

PUBLICATION INFORMATION

Full Citation: Vandenbroucke JP, Pearce N. Excess mortality calculations to assess the impact of the COVID-19 pandemic: concepts and methodological issues. *Am J Public Health*. 2024;114(6): 593–598.

Acceptance Date: December 26, 2024.

DOI: https://doi.org/10.2105/AJPH.2024.307572

CONTRIBUTORS

J. P. Vandenbroucke finalized the essay. Both authors generated the ideas for, drafted, and revised the essay.

ACKNOWLEDGMENTS

We acknowledge useful comments on a previous version by Nazrul Islam (University of Southampton, UK).

CONFLICTS OF INTEREST

The authors have no conflicts of interest to declare.

HUMAN PARTICIPANT PROTECTION

No protocol approval was necessary because data were obtained from secondary sources.

REFERENCES

1. Islam N, Shkolnikov VM, Acosta RJ, et al. Excess deaths associated with COVID-19 pandemic in 2020: age and sex disaggregated time series analysis in 29 high income countries. *BMJ*. 2021;373:n1137. https://doi.org/10.1136/bmj.n1137
2. Islam N, Jdanov DA, Shkolnikov VM, et al. Effects of COVID-19 pandemic on life expectancy and premature mortality in 2020: time series analysis in 37 countries. *BMJ*. 2021;375:e066768. https://doi.org/10.1136/bmj-2021-066768
3. Islam N. "Excess deaths" is the best metric for tracking the pandemic. *BMJ*. 2022;376:o285. https://doi.org/10.1136/bmj.o285
4. Toffolutti V, Suhrcke M. Assessing the short term health impact of the Great Recession in the European Union: a cross-country panel analysis. *Prev Med*. 2014;64:54–62. https://doi.org/10.1016/j.ypmed.2014.03.028
5. Pirkis J, John A, Shin S, et al. Suicide trends in the early months of the COVID-19 pandemic: an interrupted time-series analysis of preliminary data from 21 countries. *Lancet Psychiatry*. 2021;8(7):579–588. [Erratum in: *Lancet Psychiatry*. 2021;8(8):e18. https://doi.org/10.1016/S2215-0366(21)00213-3; Correction in: *Lancet Psychiatry*. 2021;8(11):e21. https://doi.org/10.1016/S2215-0366(21)00358-8]. https://doi.org/10.1016/S2215-0366(21)00091-2
6. Telfar-Barnard L, Baker MG, Kvalsvig A, Wilson N. COVID-19 control measure effects suggest excess winter mortality is more sensitive to infection control than warmer temperatures. *medRxiv*. 2020:2020.12.19.20248531. [Preprint: December 22, 2020]. https://doi.org/10.1101/2020.12.19.20248531
7. Oliu-Barton M, Pradelski BSR, Aghion P, et al. SARS-CoV-2 elimination, not mitigation, creates best outcomes for health, the economy, and civil liberties. *Lancet*. 2021;397(10291):2234–2236. https://doi.org/10.1016/S0140-6736(21)00978-8
8. Todd M, Scheeres A. Excess mortality from non-COVID-19 causes during the COVID-19 pandemic in Philadelphia, Pennsylvania, 2020–2021. *Am J Public Health*. 2022;112(12): 1800–1803. https://doi.org/10.2105/AJPH.2022.307096
9. Zalla LC, Mulholland GE, Filiatreau LM, Edwards JK. Racial/Ethnic and age differences in the direct and indirect effects of the COVID-19 pandemic on US mortality. *Am J Public Health*. 2022;112(1):154–164. https://doi.org/10.2105/AJPH.2021.306541
10. Galea S, Vaughan R. Tallying the ancillary consequences of COVID-19. *Am J Public Health*. 2021;111(8):1398–1399. https://doi.org/10.2105/AJPH.2021.306403
11. Kontopantelis E, Mamas MA, Webb RT, et al. Excess deaths from COVID-19 and other causes by region, neighbourhood deprivation level and place of death during the first 30 weeks of the pandemic in England and Wales: a retrospective registry study. *Lancet Reg Health Eur*. 2021;7: 100144. https://doi.org/10.1016/j.lanepe.2021
12. Cowger TL, Murray EJ, Clarke J, et al. Lifting universal masking in schools—COVID-19 incidence among students and staff. *N Engl J Med*. 2022;387(21):1935–1946. https://doi.org/10.1056/NEJMoa2211029
13. Pearce N, Vandenbroucke JP, Lawlor DA. Causal inference in environmental epidemiology: old and new approaches. *Epidemiology*. 2019; 30(3):311–316. https://doi.org/10.1097/EDE.0000000000000987
14. World Bank. Difference-in-differences. Available at: https://dimewiki.worldbank.org/Difference-in-Differences#Equal_Trends_Assumption. Accessed March 9, 2024.
15. Pearce N. Analytical implications of epidemiological concepts of interaction. *Int J Epidemiol*. 1989;18(4):976–980. https://doi.org/10.1093/ije/18.4.976
16. Pearce N, Moirano G, Maule M, et al. Does death from COVID-19 arise from a multi-step process? *Eur J Epidemiol*. 2021;36(1):1–9. https://doi.org/10.1007/s10654-020-00711-7
17. Eurostat. *Revision of the European Standard Population: Report of Eurostat's Task Force*. 2013. Available at: https://ec.europa.eu/eurostat/documents/3859598/5926869/KS-RA-13-028-EN.PDF/e713fa79-1add-44e8-b23d-5e8fa09b3f8f. Accessed March 9, 2024.
18. Bilinski A, Thompson K, Emanuel E. COVID-19 and excess all-cause mortality in the US and 20 comparison countries, June 2021–March 2022. *JAMA*. 2023;329(1):92–94. https://doi.org/10.1001/jama.2022.21795
19. Wallace J, Goldsmith-Pinkham P, Schwartz JL. Excess death rates for Republican and Democratic registered voters in Florida and Ohio during the COVID-19 pandemic. *JAMA Intern Med*. 2023;183(9):916–923. https://doi.org/10.1001/jamainternmed.2023.1154
20. Kepp KP, Bjork J, Kontis V, et al. Estimates of excess mortality for the five Nordic countries during the COVID-19 pandemic 2020–2021. *Int J Epidemiol*. 2022;51(6):1722–1732. https://doi.org/10.1093/ije/dyac204
21. Antonio-Villa NE, Bello-Chavolla OY, Fermin-Martinez CA, et al. Socio-demographic inequalities and excess non-COVID-19 mortality during the COVID-19 pandemic: a data-driven analysis of 1069174 death certificates in Mexico. *Int J Epidemiol*. 2022;51(6):1711–1721. https://doi.org/10.1093/ije/dyac184
22. Matz M, Allemani C, van Tongeren M, et al. Excess mortality among essential workers in England and Wales during the COVID-19 pandemic. *J Epidemiol Community Health*. 2022;76(7):660–666. https://doi.org/10.1136/jech-2022-218786
23. Fox MP, Murray EJ, Lesko CR, Sealy-Jefferson S. On the need to revitalize descriptive epidemiology. *Am J Epidemiol*. 2022;191(7):1174–1179. https://doi.org/10.1093/aje/kwac056

Excess Fatal Overdoses in the United States During the COVID-19 Pandemic by Geography and Substance Type: March 2020–August 2021

Jay Chandra, BA, Marie-Laure Charpignon, MS, Anushka Bhaskar, MPhil, Andrew Therriault, PhD, Yea-Hung Chen, PhD, Alyssa Mooney, PhD, Munther A. Dahleh, PhD, Mathew V. Kiang, ScD, and Francesca Dominici, PhD

See also Excess Mortality Calculations: Methods and Uses, pp. 575–609.

Objectives. To assess heterogeneity in pandemic-period excess fatal overdoses in the United States, by location (state, county) and substance type.

Methods. We used seasonal autoregressive integrated moving average (SARIMA) models to estimate counterfactual death counts in the scenario that no pandemic had occurred. Such estimates were subtracted from actual death counts to assess the magnitude of pandemic-period excess mortality between March 2020 and August 2021.

Results. Nationwide, we estimated 25 668 (95% prediction interval [PI] = 2811, 48 524) excess overdose deaths. Specifically, 17 of 47 states and 197 of 592 counties analyzed had statistically significant excess overdose-related mortality. West Virginia, Louisiana, Tennessee, Kentucky, and New Mexico had the highest rates (20–37 per 100 000). Nationally, there were 5.7 (95% PI = 1.0, 10.4), 3.1 (95% PI = 2.1, 4.2), and 1.4 (95% PI = 0.5, 2.4) excess deaths per 100 000 involving synthetic opioids, psychostimulants, and alcohol, respectively.

Conclusions. The steep increase in overdose-related mortality affected primarily the southern and western United States. We identified synthetic opioids and psychostimulants as the main contributors.

Public Health Implications. Characterizing overdose-related excess mortality across locations and substance types is critical for optimal allocation of public health resources. (*Am J Public Health*. 2024;114(6):599–609. https://doi.org/10.2105/AJPH.2024.307618)

AJPH June 2024, Vol. 114, No. 6

Over the past 20 years, fatal drug overdoses have been rising at an alarming rate in the United States.[1] A triple wave epidemic, driven by changes in substance supply and demand, has been theorized.[2] The differing characteristics of the most recent, fourth substance overdose wave underscore that this multifaceted crisis is not caused by a single substance type.[3] In particular, the surge of synthetic opioids and psychostimulant use during the COVID-19 pandemic[3] has had both important repercussions on behavioral health and implications for resource allocation, especially in rural areas of the United States.[4]

Excess mortality, defined as the discrepancy between the number of observed deaths and expected deaths, has become commonly used to understand the full burden of the pandemic.[5] This metric can retrospectively quantify the impacts of the pandemic on cause-specific deaths (e.g., cancer, diabetes, overdose).[6] Thus far, pandemic-period changes in drug overdose–related mortality have primarily been examined nationwide,[7,8] among certain racial and ethnic groups,[9–12] or in a few states or cities.[11–14]

Two studies investigated 31 states[15] and all 50 states,[16] respectively, but did not model excess mortality and instead quantified percent changes and absolute increases in drug overdose–related deaths. From a public health and policy decision-making perspective, excess-mortality approaches generally have advantages over point-in-time comparisons (i.e., percent change), including estimation of the counterfactual, acknowledgment of seasonality and long-term trends, and inclusion of uncertainty bounds.

In 2020 to 2022, 3 studies evaluated excess mortality associated with drug overdoses; they did so at the national level and for a single state (California).[7–9] County-level heterogeneity and state-level substance-specific trends in overdose mortality have yet to be studied. In addition, the extent of overdose-related excess mortality by state and of potential interactions between geography and substance type remain to be investigated. Such information could help state and local health departments allocate resources, allowing them to identify treatment needs, deploy effective outreach strategies, and implement rehabilitative and nonrehabilitative interventions that may vary with urbanicity.[17] While previous work has resulted in national recommendations—including innovation in substance use disorder treatments and disbursement methods, expansion of telehealth opportunities, enhancement of harm reduction services such as naloxone delivery, and improved access to methadone and buprenorphine,[18] such solutions may not universally apply, and their meaningful combination may depend on the location.

In this study, we quantified national-, state-, and county-level distributions of excess fatal overdoses that occurred during the pandemic, overall and for specific substance types. Each geographical unit of analysis matters; public health agencies implement prevention and recovery programs at all levels. Such a comprehensive investigation is critical for targeted resource allocation.

METHODS

Using the publicly available Centers for Disease Control and Prevention (CDC) WONDER (Wide-ranging Online Data for Epidemiologic Research) data platform,[19] we extracted cause-specific death data across all ages nationwide, by state, and by county, between January 2015 and August 2021 (see the Methods section of the Appendix, available as a supplement to the online version of this article at https://ajph.org). We identified overdose-related deaths using the underlying cause-of-death field (see the Methods section of the Appendix). The relevant *International Classification of Diseases, 10th Revision* (*ICD-10*; https://www.cdc.gov/nchs/icd/icd10.htm) codes were X40–X45 (Accidental), X60–X65 (Suicide), X85 (Homicide), and Y10–Y15 (Unknown). In addition, using the contributing cause-of-death information, we identified overdoses involving at least 1 of the following substances: heroin (T40.1), natural and semisynthetic opioids (T40.2), synthetic opioids excluding methadone (T40.4), cocaine (T40.5), psychostimulants with abuse potential (T43.6), benzodiazepines (T42.4), and alcohol (T51; Appendix Figure A).

Notably, decedents for whom the coroner or medical examiner determined the presence of multiple substances at the time of death would have certificates listing multiple contributing causes. Therefore, substance-specific categories considered in this study are not mutually exclusive, and overall overdose-related excess mortality is lower than the sum of substance-specific excess mortality. Importantly, the CDC WONDER data do not allow distinction between prescription use and illicit use. Alone, the *ICD-10* codes for underlying and contributing causes of death are insufficient to examine the potential role of substance misuse. Although partial explanations about an individual's medical history might be available in the free text section of the death certificate titled "How Injury Occurred,"[20] this part of the record may not be well-documented, even when an autopsy is performed. Moreover, the amount of details being provided about an individual's medical history and the circumstances of their death can vary substantially across medical examiners and decedents.

We estimated excess fatal overdoses both overall and by substance type by comparing observed deaths to projections based on historical trends. Our national- and overall state-level analyses capture a relatively long horizon of 18 months. Specifically, for national- and state-level estimates across all drug types, we compared counts of deaths that occurred between March 2020 and August 2021 (inclusive) to projections for this same period based on monthly data from a 5-year prepandemic period spanning January 2015 through February 2020 (inclusive). For county-level estimates across all drug types and for state-level substance-specific estimates, we similarly compared deaths that occurred in 2020 to projections based on historical data for that year. This greater level of spatial or substance type granularity required us to use yearly rather than monthly data, because of privacy-protecting data suppression in areas with few deaths in a given timeframe. For these analyses, we thus used a longer 10-year timeframe for our counterfactual models (from 2010 to 2019, inclusive). Out of 3143 counties, 592 (representing 78%

of the US population) had no missing data for 2010 to 2020 and were included in the monthly analyses; the remaining counties were excluded. Similarly, 3 states (North and South Dakota and Wyoming, representing less than 1% of the population) were excluded from the monthly analyses owing to missing data.

We used a seasonal autoregressive integrated moving average (SARIMA) model to estimate the expected number of deaths in the hypothetical scenario in which no pandemic occurred. Models were fitted separately for each substance type and geographical unit (county, state, country). Each model's parameters were chosen based on the Akaike information criterion (see Methods section in the Appendix). Once fitted to prepandemic data, the selected SARIMA model yielded projections during the pandemic period of interest, along with prediction intervals (see Methods section in the Appendix). When the observed number of deaths was outside the prediction interval (PI) for the projected number of deaths, the change in overdose-related mortality was deemed statistically significant. We conducted a sensitivity analysis to the type of model used to derive mortality projections based on prepandemic data, comparing locally estimated scatterplot smoothing models (Appendix Figure B) with the SARIMA models presented in the main analysis. We performed all analyses by using R version 4.0.2 (R Foundation for Statistical Computing, Vienna, Austria).

RESULTS

From March 2020 to August 2021, we estimated a total of 25 668 (95% PI = 2811, 48 524) excess deaths nationwide, equivalent to a mortality rate of 7.7 per 100 000 persons (95% PI = 0.9, 14.6) and 15% (95% PI = 1%, 29%) of 159 000 fatal overdoses overall. The start of the pandemic was marked by a dramatic rise in fatal overdoses: a 19% increase occurred in the 6 months that followed March 2020, relative to the counterfactual (Figure 1). Specifically, 17 out of 47 states and the District of Columbia, representing 45% of the US population, experienced a statistically significant increase in overdose-related mortality (Table 1, Figure 2). In particular, West Virginia (37 [95% PI = 2, 72] excess overdose-related deaths per 100 000), Louisiana (28; 95% PI = 16, 40), Tennessee (25; 95% PI = 18, 32), Kentucky (22; 95% PI = 1, 42), and New Mexico (20; 95% PI = 2, 38) had the highest overdose-related excess mortality rates (Table 1). These 5 states alone accounted for 21% of nationwide excess fatal overdoses (5060 in total), despite representing only 6% of the US population. These states had both high expected mortality levels and high excess mortality. Pacific coast states—including Oregon (12; 95% PI = 6, 19), Washington (11; 95% PI = 3, 18), and California (7; 95% PI = 3, 10)—also had high excess overdose-related death rates. In addition, 20 states without significant aggregate overdose-related excess mortality during the study period experienced significant excess mortality in specific months, especially either immediately following the start of the pandemic in March 2020 or 1 year later (March–May 2020 and March–May 2021).

Moreover, 197 of the 592 counties analyzed, representing 36% of the US population, had a statistically significant increase in overdose-related mortality in 2020 (Figure 3, Appendix Table A). Among the 50 counties with the highest overdose-related excess mortality, half were located in the 5 most-affected states. Geographical clustering was notable: the 4 counties with the largest excess mortality rates (65–78 excess deaths per 100 000) were all located in West Virginia. Many of these counties had both high expected drug overdose–related deaths and high excess mortality (Appendix Figure C). However, we also identified a few outlying counties with high excess mortality in states that overall did not exhibit such a pattern (e.g., Monroe County, Pennsylvania; see the Results section of the Appendix). Our results also highlighted county-level differences based on urbanicity, but with variations across states as illustrated by the case of Florida versus Texas (see the Results section of the Appendix).

Importantly, national-level excess overdose-related mortality also varied across substance types. The primary contributors were synthetic opioids (5.7 [95% PI = 1.0, 10.4] excess deaths per 100 000; 18 782), psychostimulants (3.1; 95% PI = 2.1, 4.2; 10 345), and alcohol poisoning (1.4; 95% PI = 0.5, 2.4; 4797; Figure 1, Appendix Figure D). Of the 50 states and DC, 40 (representing 95% of the US population) had statistically significant excess mortality involving synthetic opioids. In addition, mortality rates linked to psychostimulants, benzodiazepines, cocaine, and alcohol significantly exceeded projections in 29, 20, 18, and 18 states, respectively. However, mortality rates associated with heroin as well as with natural and semisynthetic opioids rose significantly in only 4 and 7 states, respectively. Interestingly, New York was one of the rare states significantly affected by both heroin (1.1 [95% PI = 0.2, 2.1] excess deaths per 100 000) and natural and semisynthetic opioids (1.4; 95% PI = 0.3, 2.6). West Virginia had the highest excess mortality for all

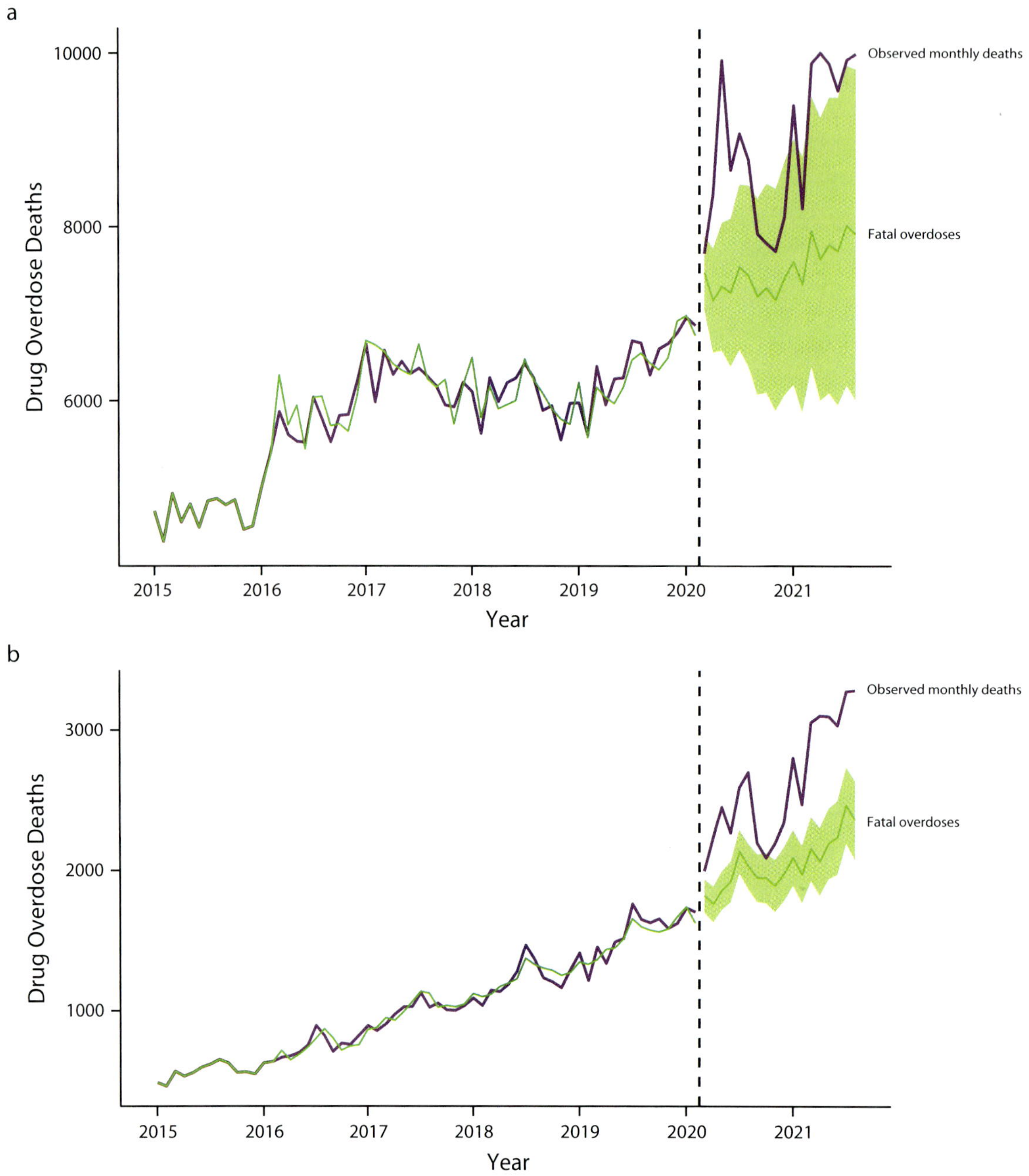

FIGURE 1— Observed and Projected Overdose Mortality From (a) All Substance Types and (b) Psychostimulants: United States, March 2020–August 2021 (Inclusive)

Note. Substance-specific overdose mortality involving synthetic opioids, cocaine, heroin, benzodiazepines, natural and semisynthetic opioids, and alcohol are displayed in Appendix Figure D (available as a supplement to the online version of this article at https://ajph.org). The substance-specific categories are not mutually exclusive. Purple lines represent observed monthly deaths; green lines represent the fitted and projected fatal overdoses based on counterfactual estimates derived from prepandemic data (Jan 2015–Feb 2020) using a seasonal auto-regressive integrated moving average model. Dashed vertical line indicates transition between prepandemic and pandemic period, defined as starting on Mar 1, 2020. Shaded green area, during the pandemic period, corresponds to 95% prediction interval (PI) for absolute number of fatal overdoses at the national level, from Mar 2020–Aug 2021. The difference between the purple line and the green line to the right of the dashed line is the estimated excess mortality. The difference between the purple line and the lower and upper bounds of the PI results in a PI for excess mortality.

TABLE 1— Estimates of Overall Excess Fatal Overdoses for 47 US States and the District of Columbia: March 2020–August 2021, (Inclusive)

State	Expected No. of Fatal Overdoses (95% PI)	Observed No. of Fatal Overdoses	Ratio (Observed/ Expected)	Excess Deaths, No. (95% PI)	Excess Deaths per 100 000 Persons, No. (95% PI)	COVID-19 Deaths per 100 000 Persons, No.
US overall[a]	135 191 (112 334, 158 048)	160 859	1.19	25 668 (2 811, 48 524)	7.7 (0.9, 14.6)	181
Alabama[a]	1 318 (802, 1 833)	1 904	1.45	586 (71, 1102)	11.7 (1.4, 21.9)	252
Alaska	253 (112, 394)	354	1.40	101 (−40, 242)	13.8 (−5.5, 33)	62
Arizona	3 916 (3 088, 4 744)	4 523	1.16	607 (−221, 1 435)	8.5 (−3.1, 20.1)	217
Arkansas	858 (504, 1 211)	962	1.12	104 (−249, 458)	3.5 (−8.3, 15.2)	222
California[a]	13 496 (12 110, 14 883)	16 161	1.20	2 665 (1 278, 4 051)	6.7 (3.2, 10.2)	164
Colorado[a]	2 257 (1 751, 2 763)	2 849	1.26	592 (86, 1098)	10.3 (1.5, 19.0)	110
Connecticut	2 239 (1 585, 2 892)	2 239	1.00	0 (−653, 654)	0.0 (−18.1, 18.1)	214
Delaware	797 (520, 1 074)	723	0.91	−74 (−351, 203)	−7.5 (−35.4, 20.5)	168
District of Columbia	735 (282, 1 187)	656	0.89	−79 (−531, 374)	−11.4 (−77.1, 54.2)	171
Florida	10 363 (7 359, 13 367)	11 876	1.15	1 513 (−1 491, 4 517)	7.0 (−6.9, 21.0)	197
Georgia[a]	2 451 (1 745, 3 157)	3 468	1.42	1 017 (311, 1 723)	9.5 (2.9, 16.1)	180
Hawaii	414 (245, 582)	450	1.09	36 (−132, 205)	2.5 (−9.1, 14.1)	44
Idaho	462 (274, 650)	510	1.10	48 (−140, 236)	2.6 (−7.6, 12.8)	116
Illinois	5 738 (3 726, 7 750)	5 751	1.00	13 (−1 999, 2 025)	0.1 (−15.6, 15.8)	174
Indiana	3 522 (2 502, 4 542)	4 132	1.17	610 (−410, 1 630)	9.0 (−6.0, 24.0)	184
Iowa	823 (529, 1 117)	799	0.97	−24 (−318, 270)	−0.7 (−10, 8.5)	178
Kansas	768 (516, 1 020)	987	1.29	219 (−33, 471)	7.5 (−1.1, 16.0)	179
Kentucky[a]	2 605 (1 665, 3 544)	3 578	1.37	973 (34, 1 913)	21.6 (0.8, 42.5)	170
Louisiana[a]	2 330 (1 778, 2 883)	3 623	1.55	1 293 (740, 1 845)	27.8 (15.9, 39.6)	236
Maine	793 (409, 1 177)	813	1.03	20 (−364, 404)	1.5 (−26.7, 29.7)	70
Maryland	3 655 (2 138, 5 173)	4 396	1.20	741 (−777, 2 258)	12.0 (−12.6, 36.6)	153
Massachusetts	3 597 (2 463, 4 731)	3 759	1.05	162 (−972, 1 296)	2.3 (−13.8, 18.4)	179
Michigan	3 921 (2 384, 5 459)	4 548	1.16	627 (−911, 2 164)	6.2 (−9.0, 21.5)	175
Minnesota[a]	1 340 (958, 1 723)	1 944	1.45	604 (221, 986)	10.6 (3.9, 17.3)	122
Mississippi[a]	584 (352, 816)	1 089	1.86	505 (273, 737)	17.1 (9.2, 24.9)	269
Missouri	3 121 (2 353, 3 890)	3 453	1.11	332 (−437, 1 100)	5.4 (−7.1, 17.9)	194
Montana	242 (114, 371)	296	1.22	54 (−75, 182)	4.9 (−6.9, 16.8)	149
Nebraska	288 (167, 410)	381	1.32	93 (−29, 214)	4.7 (−1.5, 10.9)	139
Nevada[a]	1 194 (855, 1 532)	1 583	1.33	389 (51, 728)	12.5 (1.6, 23.4)	205
New Hampshire	588 (241, 936)	626	1.06	38 (−310, 385)	2.7 (−22.5, 28.0)	95
New Jersey	5 132 (3 251, 7 012)	4 530	0.88	−602 (−2482, 1279)	−6.5 (−26.7, 13.8)	245
New Mexico[a]	1 183 (789, 1 577)	1 584	1.34	401 (7, 795)	18.9 (0.3, 37.5)	205
New York	7 140 (5 391, 8 889)	8 271	1.16	1 131 (−618, 2 880)	5.6 (−3.1, 14.3)	256
North Carolina	4 227 (3 019, 5 436)	5 411	1.28	1 184 (−25, 2 392)	11.3 (−0.2, 22.9)	154
Ohio	7 182 (3 981, 10 384)	8 649	1.20	1 467 (−1735, 4 668)	12.4 (−14.7, 39.6)	182
Oklahoma	1 110 (522, 1 697)	1 484	1.34	374 (−213, 962)	9.5 (−5.4, 24.3)	234
Oregon[a]	1 035 (762, 1 309)	1 555	1.50	520 (246, 793)	12.3 (5.8, 18.7)	73
Pennsylvania	7 532 (3 283, 11 780)	8 317	1.10	785 (−3 463, 5 034)	6.0 (−26.6, 38.7)	201
Rhode Island	496 (305, 687)	646	1.30	150 (−41, 341)	13.7 (−3.7, 31.0)	204
South Carolina[a]	2 183 (1 553, 2 812)	2 991	1.37	808 (179, 1 438)	15.8 (3.5, 28.1)	207

Continued

AJPH June 2024, Vol. 114, No. 6

TABLE 1— Continued

State	Expected No. of Fatal Overdoses (95% PI)	Observed No. of Fatal Overdoses	Ratio (Observed/ Expected)	Excess Deaths, No. (95% PI)	Excess Deaths per 100 000 Persons, No. (95% PI)	COVID-19 Deaths per 100 000 Persons, No.
Tennessee[a]	3 713 (3 217, 4 208)	5 420	1.46	1 707 (1 212, 2 203)	24.7 (17.5, 31.9)	191
Texas[a]	6 224 (5 198, 7 250)	7 788	1.25	1 564 (538, 2 590)	5.4 (1.8, 8.9)	203
Utah	843 (323, 1 363)	1 063	1.26	220 (−300, 740)	6.7 (−9.2, 22.6)	74
Vermont	289 (125, 454)	349	1.21	60 (−105, 224)	9.3 (−16.3, 34.9)	37
Virginia[a]	2 692 (1 833, 3 550)	3 738	1.39	1 046 (188, 1 905)	12.1 (2.2, 22.1)	129
Washington[a]	2 405 (1 795, 3 015)	3 215	1.34	810 (200, 1 420)	10.5 (2.6, 18.4)	75
West Virginia[a]	1 669 (1 047, 2 291)	2 330	1.40	661 (39, 1 283)	36.9 (2.2, 71.5)	169
Wisconsin	2 295 (1 580, 3 009)	2 568	1.12	273 (−441, 988)	4.6 (−7.5, 16.8)	126

Note. PI = prediction interval. Additional information about the calculation of point estimates and prediction intervals is provided in the Methods section of the Appendix (available as a supplement to the online version of this article at https://ajph.org). There were no statistically significant decreases. Three states (ND, SD, and WY), representing less than 1% of the US population, were excluded from the analysis owing to missing data: the CDC WONDER platform does not return any value for cells with a death count strictly lower than 10.
[a]States with statistically significant increases (n = 17).

AJPH June 2024, Vol. 114, No. 6

substances, except cocaine, for which Rhode Island was the most-affected state. The states most affected by cocaine-related excess mortality were primarily located in the central and northeastern parts of the country, in addition to Alaska and Hawaii.

The geographical distribution of psychostimulant-, benzodiazepine-, and alcohol-related overdose excess mortality followed the pattern of overall overdose-related excess mortality, with the addition of a few states in the Northeast (New York, Rhode Island, Pennsylvania) and Midwest (Nebraska, Wisconsin). Despite having nonsignificant excess mortality overall, Rhode Island had the fourth highest excess mortality rate related to synthetic opioids in the country (9.1 [95% PI = 5.8, 12.4] per 100 000). Vermont also had low excess fatal overdoses overall but significantly high excess mortality involving synthetic opioids (7.0 [95% PI = 2.8, 11.2] per 100 000), cocaine (4.0 [95% PI = 2.4, 5.6] per 100 000), and benzodiazepines (3.7 [95% PI = 1.2, 6.3] per 100 000). Additional visualizations and tables displaying substance-specific results are provided at https://github.com/jaychandra3/Drug_Overdose.

Furthermore, the repercussions of the COVID-19 pandemic on overdose-related mortality shifted over time. While excess mortality during the longer pandemic period spanning March 2020 to August 2021 was significant only for synthetic opioids, psychostimulants, and alcohol, the initial peak in fatal overdoses observed in May 2020 was unambiguous and affected all substance types (Figure 1, Appendix Figure D). Indeed, we found considerable excess mortality across all substance types during the first 3 months of the pandemic (March–May 2020), marking a clear divergence from prepandemic trends: increases were statistically significant for synthetic opioids (1.0 [95% PI = 0.7, 1.4] excess deaths per 100 000), cocaine (0.3; 95% PI = 0.1, 0.4), psychostimulants (0.4; 95% PI = 0.3, 0.5), benzodiazepines (0.3; 95% PI = 0.1, 0.4), alcohol (0.2; 95% PI = 0.1, 0.3), heroin (0.1; 95% PI = 0, 0.3), and natural and semisynthetic opioids (0.1; 95% PI = 0.0, 0.2). Following this 3-month period, overdose deaths involving benzodiazepines, natural and semisynthetic opioids, and cocaine returned nearly to the levels projected using prepandemic trends, while heroin overdose deaths dropped below projections. In contrast, fatal overdoses involving alcohol, psychostimulants, or synthetic opioids continued to outpace projections during the remainder of the 18-month study period, stressing the mid- to long-term effects of the pandemic on overdose-related absolute and excess mortality (Figure 1).

DISCUSSION

The steep increase in fatal overdoses in the months following March 2020 may indicate the rapid, substantial effect of the COVID-19 pandemic on substance use, especially in southern and Pacific coast states. Most previous work published in

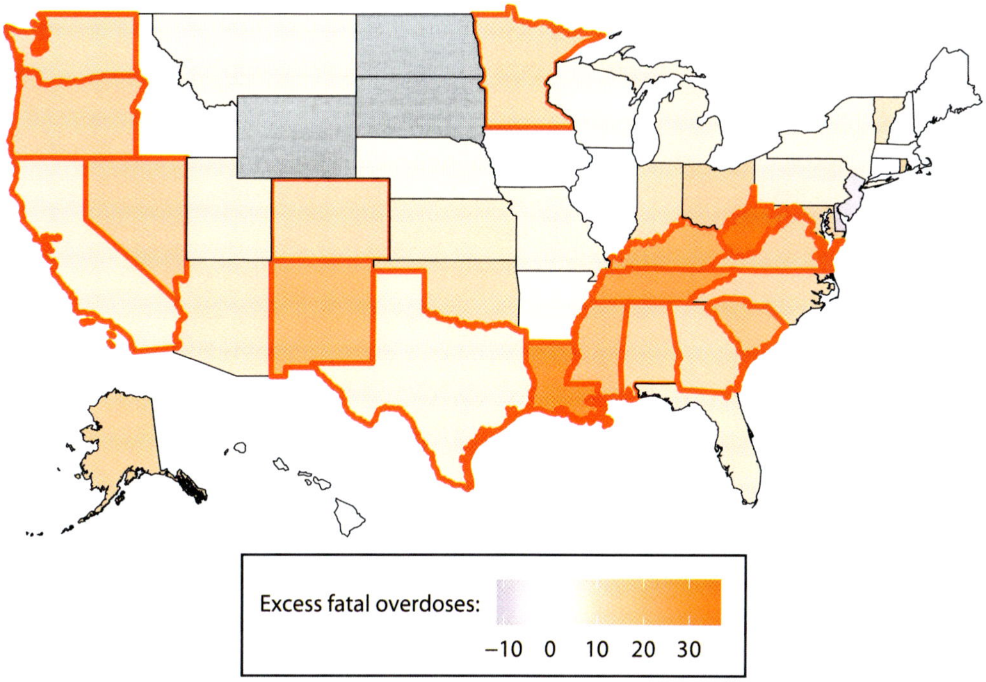

FIGURE 2— **Excess Fatal Overdoses by State: United States, March 2020–August 2021 (Inclusive)**

Note. States in gray (n = 3) lacked sufficient data for estimation. States with orange boundaries (n = 17) had a statistically significant increase in overdose-related mortality between Mar 2020 and Aug 2021. States in orange (n = 44) had an increase in overdose-related mortality (relative to the counterfactual). States in purple (n = 4) had a non–statistically significant decrease in overdose-related mortality.

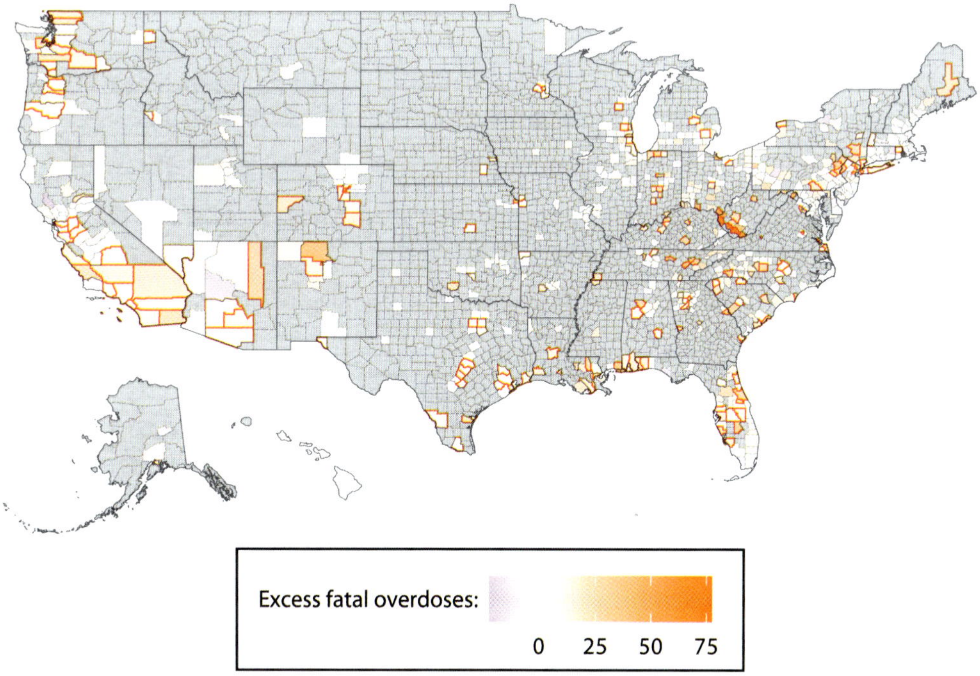

FIGURE 3— **Excess Fatal Overdoses by County: United States, 2020**

Note. Counties in gray (n = 2551) lacked sufficient data for estimation. Counties with orange boundaries (n = 197) had positive and statistically significant excess overdose-related mortality in 2020. Counties in orange (n = 487) had positive excess overdose-related mortality. Counties in purple (n = 105) had negative excess overdose-related mortality.

2020 to 2022 has analyzed overdose-related mortality at the national level only.[7,8] While examining macro-trends in substance-related mortality is important for nationwide public health decision-making, local analyses also matter as they provide valuable insights for tailored interventions. Our study acknowledges this trade-off by adopting a dual focus. Through modeling of absolute and excess fatal overdoses across US states and counties as well as by substance, our study expands upon previous research by analyzing nationwide trends by substance and demonstrating the importance of granular geographical characterization for postpandemic resource (re)allocation.

Future work could involve the development and implementation of methods to explicitly account for similarities among geographically proximal units. Notably, in 2019, Haffajee et al. had proposed a method to identify counties with high opioid overdose mortality, arguing that it could help target support programs toward areas with the greatest needs.[21] Following the pandemic shock, it is important to revisit this approach to account for changes in regional demographics and health behaviors, which are critical for resource allocation.[22] By contrasting prepandemic and pandemic-period fatal overdoses by substance type, we provide new information to assist with identifying high-risk counties. Resource allocation based solely on state-level data or ignoring yearly adjustments might overlook highly vulnerable counties. As an example, we show that individual counties in a given state can appear as outliers and present high excess mortality despite the state having low excess mortality in aggregate, underscoring the extent of geographical heterogeneity. The opposite pattern can also appear (i.e., states with high excess mortality overall but with counties that are not severely affected).

For public health officials, the geographical granularity of our study allows identification of adjacent counties that may benefit from pooling their resources. Quantifying the distributions of substance-specific overdose deaths among counties and states and pandemic-period shifts can also inform program design. We show that while almost all states had significant excess mortality associated with synthetic opioids, other substance types affected only specific regions or a small subset of states (e.g., cocaine: central and northeastern United States; heroin: Iowa, Georgia, South Carolina, and New York).

We hypothesize that several factors may have interacted and differentially affected certain states or counties owing to place-based, structural socioeconomic factors[23] and dynamic evolutions of the epidemic and labor market. First, the overburdened health system may have resulted in decreased attention to overdose-related morbidity and mortality. This burden has been primarily linked to synthetic opioids and psychostimulants. The growing availability of highly potent drugs such as fentanyl has largely contributed to drug overdose–related excess mortality,[24,25] but distinct geographical patterns have emerged, including greater involvement of psychostimulants in rural versus urban overdose deaths.[26]

Second, in regard to changes in socio-behavioral factors, the pandemic may have worsened individual-level correlates of substance use and risk of overdose, such as mental health issues, social isolation, and homelessness.[27] Survey respondents have reported that growing anxiety and lack of employment made them more likely to use drugs alone than before the pandemic, a setting that can, in turn, increase the risk of overdose.[28] The consumption of drugs or alcohol as a stress-induced coping mechanism[29] might explain the sudden increase in fatal overdoses, especially among individuals facing substance use disorder for the first time during the pandemic. Notably, we found that alcohol-related overdose deaths consistently outpaced projections over the considered time period, corroborating a previous study.[30] For relapsing individuals, shifts in lifestyle and economic insecurity may have compounded with limited access to substance use disorder treatment and support services.[31] The perception of changes to service provisions might also have increased self-stigma,[32] thereby lowering health care utilization. Further research is needed to elucidate the underlying socio-behavioral contexts and their interaction with biological and environmental factors.

Lastly, a decline in heroin-related overdose mortality was initiated in 2017. This prepandemic trend may in part explain the patterns we have observed over the study period, along with pandemic-period changes in supply and demand. Mobility restrictions, long-lasting border closures, and declines in world trade that affected global supply chains during the pandemic all significantly disrupted drug supply.[33] Indeed, most heroin and cocaine imports from Mexico, Colombia, Peru, and Southwest Asia[34] may have been substituted by either toxic and adulterated substances or by more potent drugs such as fentanyl, thereby amplifying the risk of fatal overdose.[35] Empirical evidence from surveys and qualitative interviews confirms that several factors contributed to increased exposure to fentanyl, including the scarcity of heroin, increasing cost of methamphetamine, and emergence of inexpensive fentanyl-derived products.[36] A rising number of fatalities have been attributed to counterfeit pills and heroin mixed with fentanyl, which could be transported in much smaller quantities when cross-border mobility was limited by border restrictions. This reality was more pronounced in regions close to Mexico.[37] In September 2023, a CDC report[38] quantified the impact: evidence of counterfeit pill use in overdose deaths more than doubled between July to September 2019 and October to December 2021 (from 2.0% to 4.7% of overall overdose deaths), and tripled in western US states (from 4.7% to 14.7%). Further research is needed to causally identify the relative contribution of increases in counterfeit pill supply on fatal overdoses.

Limitations

This study has 4 main limitations. First, death projections based on prepandemic trends are assumed to be valid counterfactuals from which excess mortality estimates are derived. The goodness-of-fit evaluation of our models resulted in a mean absolute percentage error (MAPE) of only 8% across the 47 considered states with a minimum MAPE of 3% (California) and a maximum MAPE of 17% (Delaware). For 90% of states (42 out of 47), the MAPE was lower than 13%. However, projections based on fluctuating levels of prepandemic mortality can be difficult to obtain in certain locations (e.g., Ohio, Pennsylvania). Furthermore, whether the increase or decrease in death counts is linear, polynomial, or exponential may be challenging to determine in certain states (e.g., California, Florida). Such uncertainties can yield wider PIs. Consequently, statistical significance is generally conservative in this study. Furthermore, the nonstatistical significance of excess mortality estimates in certain states (e.g., Rhode Island, Alaska) may owe in part to small population sizes and highly variable overdose-related mortality rates during the prepandemic period.

Despite this first limitation, our results about pandemic-period excess fatal overdoses seem robust to model choice. In sensitivity analyses involving models that overweigh proximal points and tend to project exponential rather than linear growth, the roster of states with significant overdose-related mortality was similar to that of the main analysis (76% overlap, see Methods section of the Appendix). Moreover, we confirmed that our model did not estimate significant excess mortality in any state before the pandemic (see Methods section of the Appendix). This validation provides further evidence that the magnitude of overdose-related excess mortality is strongly associated with the pandemic rather than an artifact of poor model fit.

Second, there are limitations associated with the reporting of causes of death in vital records. The heterogeneity in fatal overdoses observed across states might be influenced by differing practices among coroners and medical examiners. The quality of death certificate data can also vary over time as reporting practices and incentives evolve.[39] Additionally, toxicology assessments may not be conducted systematically, yielding variation in the proportion of death certificates with an "unknown/unspecified" drug code (T50.9) across states.[39] For instance, investigating the presence of fentanyl requires a second toxicology assessment, which incurs additional costs. Therefore, substance-specific excess mortality estimates presented in our study reflect only death certificates in which specific overdose-related labels are present. More efforts are needed to mitigate missing or poor-quality data in vital records.

Third, our study relied exclusively on *ICD-10* codes reported on death certificates and data queries from the CDC WONDER online platform. Thus, it does not allow examination of substance misuse. Going forward, an analysis attempting to link electronic health records or claims data with death certificates at the county or even zip code level may be warranted to learn more about the role of prescription drug use on excess mortality, identify any geographical differences, and potentially implement targeted interventions.

Fourth, in the present study, we have investigated differences in overdose-related excess mortality rates by age group across states only overall. Next, we plan to additionally study the 3-way interaction among substance type, geography, and socio-demographics (including age). In the future, the broader objective is to work closely with state departments of public health to allow for near-real-time monitoring of excess mortality patterns.

Conclusions

Overall, the COVID-19 pandemic had a disparate impact on overdose-related mortality. Our granular geographical analysis of the burden has identified areas that were more affected than others, including outlying counties. Furthermore, our work has revealed the emergence of new patterns by substance type and the increasing involvement of alcohol in overdose deaths. To complement the national recommendations of the Stanford-Lancet Commission for the North American Opioid Crisis,[18] we encourage the CDC to tailor public health messaging by geography and local departments of health to strengthen existing death investigation systems to characterize with precision the socioeconomic, psychosocial, and pharmacological needs of their populations. We hope our results will drive additional research into the state-specific mechanisms by which the pandemic and the substance overdose crisis interact and prompt changes to resource allocation to prevent overdose deaths in the most vulnerable communities. AJPH

ABOUT THE AUTHORS

Jay Chandra is with Harvard Medical School, Harvard University, Boston, MA. Marie-Laure Charpignon and Munther A. Dahleh are with the Institute for Data, Systems, and Society, Massachusetts Institute of Technology, Cambridge. Anushka Bhaskar and Andrew Therriault are with the Department of Government, Harvard University, Cambridge. Yea-Hung Chen is with the Department of Epidemiology and Biostatistics, University of California, San Francisco. Alyssa Mooney is with the Institute for Health Policy Studies, University of California, San Francisco. Mathew V. Kiang is with the Department of Epidemiology and Population Health, Stanford University, Stanford, CA. Francesca Dominici is with the Department of Biostatistics, T.H. Chan School of Public Health, Harvard University, Boston.

CORRESPONDENCE

Correspondence should be sent to Jay Chandra, 107 Avenue Louis Pasteur, Boston, MA 02115 (e-mail: jay_chandra@hms.harvard.edu). Reprints can be ordered at https://ajph.org by clicking the "Reprints" link.

PUBLICATION INFORMATION

Full Citation: Chandra J, Charpignon M-L, Bhaskar A, et al. Excess fatal overdoses in the United States during the COVID-19 pandemic by geography and substance type: March 2020–August 2021. *Am J Public Health*. 2024;114(6):599–609.

Acceptance Date: January 26, 2024.

DOI: https://doi.org/10.2105/AJPH.2024.307618

CONTRIBUTORS

J. Chandra and M.-L. Charpignon equally contributed to this work. J. Chandra and A. Bhaskar participated in the conceptualization of the study, formal analysis, methodology, validation, and visualization. M.-L. Charpignon participated in the conceptualization of the study, formal analysis, methodology, project administration, validation, and visualization. A. Therriault participated in the conceptualization of the study and methodology. Y.-H. Chen participated in the methodology and supervision. M.A. Dahleh participated in the supervision. M.V. Kiang and F. Dominici participated in the methodology, project administration, and supervision. All authors participated in writing the original draft, reviewed and edited the article, and have read and agreed to the published version of the article. Mathew V. Kiang and Francesca Dominici were co-senior authors.

CONFLICTS OF INTEREST

We have no conflicts of interest to disclose.

HUMAN PARTICIPANT PROTECTION

This study used publicly available data and was not subject to human participant protection review at Harvard or the Massachusetts Institute of Technology.

REFERENCES

1. Hedegaard H, Miniño AM, Spencer MR, Warner M. Drug overdose deaths in the United States, 1999–2020. *NCHS Data Brief*. 2021;(426):1–8. https://doi.org/10.15620/cdc:112340
2. Ciccarone D. The triple wave epidemic: supply and demand drivers of the US opioid overdose crisis. *Int J Drug Policy*. 2019;71:183–188. https://doi.org/10.1016/j.drugpo.2019.01.010
3. Fischer B, O'Keefe-Markman C, Lee AMH, Daldegan-Bueno D. "Resurgent," "twin" or "silent" epidemic? A select data overview and observations on increasing psycho-stimulant use and harms in North America. *Subst Abuse Treat Prev Policy*. 2021;16(1):17. https://doi.org/10.1186/s13011-021-00350-5
4. Manchikanti L, Singh VM, Staats PS, et al. Fourth wave of opioid (illicit drug) overdose deaths and diminishing access to prescription opioids and interventional techniques: cause and effect. *Pain Physician*. 2022;25(2):97–124.
5. Beaney T, Clarke JM, Jain V, et al. Excess mortality: the gold standard in measuring the impact of COVID-19 worldwide? *J R Soc Med*. 2020;113(9):329–334. https://doi.org/10.1177/0141076820956802
6. Woolf SH, Chapman DA, Sabo RT, Zimmerman EB. Excess deaths from COVID-19 and other causes in the US, March 1, 2020, to January 2, 2021. *JAMA*. 2021;325(17):1786–1789. https://doi.org/10.1001/jama.2021.5199
7. Cartus AR, Li Y, Macmadu A, et al. Forecasted and observed drug overdose deaths in the US during the COVID-19 pandemic in 2020. *JAMA Netw Open*. 2022;5(3):e223418. https://doi.org/10.1001/jamanetworkopen.2022.3418
8. Faust JS, Du C, Mayes KD, et al. Mortality from drug overdoses, homicides, unintentional injuries, motor vehicle crashes, and suicides during the pandemic, March–August 2020. *JAMA*. 2021;326(1):84–86. https://doi.org/10.1001/jama.2021.8012
9. Kiang MV, Acosta RJ, Chen YH, et al. Sociodemographic and geographic disparities in excess fatal drug overdoses during the COVID-19 pandemic in California: a population-based study. *Lancet Reg Health Am*. 2022;11:100237. https://doi.org/10.1016/j.lana.2022.100237
10. Han B, Einstein EB, Jones CM, Cotto J, Compton WM, Volkow ND. Racial and ethnic disparities in drug overdose deaths in the US during the COVID-19 pandemic. *JAMA Netw Open*. 2022;5(9):e2232314. https://doi.org/10.1001/jamanetworkopen.2022.32314
11. Macmadu A, Batthala S, Correia Gabel AM, et al. Comparison of characteristics of deaths from drug overdose before vs during the COVID-19 pandemic in Rhode Island. *JAMA Netw Open*. 2021;4(9):e2125538. https://doi.org/10.1001/jamanetworkopen.2021.25538
12. Kelley MA, Lucas J, Stewart E, Goldman D, Doctor JN. Opioid-related deaths before and after COVID-19 stay-at-home orders in Los Angeles County. *Drug Alcohol Depend*. 2021;228:109028. https://doi.org/10.1016/j.drugalcdep.2021.109028
13. Currie JM, Schnell MK, Schwandt H, Zhang J. Trends in drug overdose mortality in Ohio during the first 7 months of the COVID-19 pandemic. *JAMA Netw Open*. 2021;4(4):e217112. https://doi.org/10.1001/jamanetworkopen.2021.7112
14. Slavova S, Quesinberry D, Hargrove S, et al. Trends in drug overdose mortality rates in Kentucky, 2019–2020. *JAMA Netw Open*. 2021;4(7):e2116391. https://doi.org/10.1001/jamanetworkopen.2021.16391
15. Friedman J, Akre S. COVID-19 and the drug overdose crisis: uncovering the deadliest months in the United States, January–July 2020. *Am J Public Health*. 2021;111(7):1284–1291. https://doi.org/10.2105/AJPH.2021.306256
16. Chen C, Shen S. Trend analysis of drug overdose deaths before and during the COVID-19 pandemic. *Am J Transl Res*. 2022;14(4):2685–2688.
17. Post LA, Lundberg A, Moss CB, et al. Geographic trends in opioid overdoses in the US from 1999 to 2020. *JAMA Netw Open*. 2022;5(7):e2223631. https://doi.org/10.1001/jamanetworkopen.2022.23631
18. Humphreys K, Shover CL, Andrews CM, et al. Responding to the opioid crisis in North America and beyond: recommendations of the Stanford-Lancet Commission. *Lancet*. 2022;399(10324):555–604. https://doi.org/10.1016/S0140-6736(21)02252-2
19. CDC WONDER. Available at: https://wonder.cdc.gov. Accessed December 1, 2022.
20. Davis GG, Cadwallader AB, Fligner CL, et al. Position paper: recommendations for the investigation, diagnosis, and certification of deaths related to opioid and other drugs. *Am J Forensic Med Pathol*. 2020;41(3):152–159. https://doi.org/10.1097/PAF.0000000000000550
21. Haffajee RL, Lin LA, Bohnert ASB, Goldstick JE. Characteristics of US counties with high opioid overdose mortality and low capacity to deliver medications for opioid use disorder. *JAMA Netw Open*. 2019;2(6):e196373. https://doi.org/10.1001/jamanetworkopen.2019.6373

22. Evans AC. The critical need for a population health approach: addressing the nation's behavioral health during the COVID-19 pandemic and beyond. *Prev Chronic Dis.* 2020;17:200261. https://doi.org/10.5888/pcd17.200261
23. Monnat SM, Peters DJ, Berg MT, Hochstetler A. Using census data to understand county-level differences in overall drug mortality and opioid-related mortality by opioid type. *Am J Public Health.* 2019;109(8):1084–1091. https://doi.org/10.2105/AJPH.2019.305136
24. Mattson CL. Trends and geographic patterns in drug and synthetic opioid overdose deaths—United States, 2013–2019. *MMWR Morb Mortal Wkly Rep.* 2021;70(6):202–207. https://doi.org/10.15585/mmwr.mm7006a4
25. Han B, Compton WM, Jones CM, Einstein EB, Volkow ND. Methamphetamine use, methamphetamine use disorder, and associated overdose deaths among US adults. *JAMA Psychiatry.* 2021;78(12):1329–1342. https://doi.org/10.1001/jamapsychiatry.2021.2588
26. Hedegaard H, Miniño AM, Warner M. Urban–rural differences in drug overdose death rates, by sex, age, and type of drugs involved, 2017. *NCHS Data Brief.* 2019:(345):1–8.
27. Stanford S, Raja K, Pegna SW, et al. Identifying the root causes of drug overdose health inequities and related social determinants of health: a literature review. Centers for Disease Control and Prevention. August 2021. Available at: https://stacks.cdc.gov/view/cdc/114435. Accessed December 20, 2023.
28. Walters SM, Bolinski RS, Almirol E, et al. Structural and community changes during COVID-19 and their effects on overdose precursors among rural people who use drugs: a mixed-methods analysis. *Addict Sci Clin Pract.* 2022;17(1):24. https://doi.org/10.1186/s13722-022-00303-8
29. Pedrosa AL, Bitencourt L, Fróes ACF, et al. Emotional, behavioral, and psychological impact of the COVID-19 pandemic. *Front Psychol.* 2020;11:566212. https://doi.org/10.3389/fpsyg.2020.566212
30. White AM, Castle IJP, Powell PA, Hingson RW, Koob GF. Alcohol-related deaths during the COVID-19 pandemic. *JAMA.* 2022;327(17):1704–1706. https://doi.org/10.1001/jama.2022.4308
31. Zvolensky MJ, Garey L, Rogers AH, et al. Psychological, addictive, and health behavior implications of the COVID-19 pandemic. *Behav Res Ther.* 2020;134:103715. https://doi.org/10.1016/j.brat.2020.103715
32. Dannatt L, Ransing R, Calvey T, et al. The impact of stigma on treatment services for people with substance use disorders during the COVID-19 pandemic—perspectives of NECPAM members. *Front Psychiatry.* 2021;12:634515. https://doi.org/10.3389/fpsyt.2021.634515
33. United Nations Office on Drugs and Crime. COVID-19 and the drug supply chain: from production and trafficking to use. Available at: https://www.emcdda.europa.eu/drugs-library/covid-19-and-drug-supply-chain-production-and-trafficking-use-unodc_en. Accessed December 20, 2023.
34. Atkinson S. Toward developing estimates of US imports of illegal drugs. US Bureau of Economic Analysis. February 2020. Available at: https://www.bea.gov/research/papers/2020/toward-developing-estimates-us-imports-illegal-drugs. Accessed April 28, 2023.
35. Ali F, Russell C, Nafeh F, Rehm J, LeBlanc S, Elton-Marshall T. Changes in substance supply and use characteristics among people who use drugs (PWUD) during the COVID-19 global pandemic: a national qualitative assessment in Canada. *Int J Drug Policy.* 2021;93:103237. https://doi.org/10.1016/j.drugpo.2021.103237
36. Bolinski RS, Walters S, Salisbury-Afshar E, et al. The impact of the COVID-19 pandemic on drug use behaviors, fentanyl exposure, and harm reduction service support among people who use drugs in rural settings. *Int J Environ Res Public Health.* 2022;19(4):2230. https://doi.org/10.3390/ijerph19042230
37. Friedman J, Godvin M, Molina C, et al. Fentanyl, heroin, and methamphetamine-based counterfeit pills sold at tourist-oriented pharmacies in Mexico: an ethnographic and drug checking study. *Drug Alcohol Depend.* 2023:249:110819. https://doi.org/10.1016/j.drugalcdep.2023.110819.
38. O'Donnell J. Drug overdose deaths with evidence of counterfeit pill use—United States, July 2019–December 2021. *MMWR Morb Mortal Wkly Rep.* 2023;72(35):949–956. https://doi.org/10.15585/mmwr.mm7235a3
39. Warner M, Paulozzi LJ, Nolte KB, Davis GG, Nelson LS. State variation in certifying manner of death and drugs involved in drug intoxication deaths. *Academic Forensic Pathology.* 2013;3(2):231–237. https://doi.org/10.23907/2013.029

First Decade of Supportive Services for Veteran Families Program and Homelessness, 2012–2022

Renae Wilkinson, PhD, Thomas Byrne, PhD, Richard G. Cowden, PhD, Katelyn N.G. Long, DrPH, MSc, John H. Kuhn, MPH, Howard K. Koh, MD, MPH, and Jack Tsai, PhD, MSCP

See also Bamberger, p. 548.

As homelessness remains an urgent public health crisis in the United States, specific programs in the US Department of Veterans Affairs (VA) system may serve as a roadmap for addressing it.

We examine lessons learned from the first decade (2012–2022) of the Supportive Services for Veteran Families (SSVF) program, a cornerstone in the VA continuum of homeless services aimed at both preventing homelessness among those at risk and providing rapid rehousing for veterans and their families who are currently experiencing homelessness. Drawing on information from annual reports and other relevant literature, we have identified 3 themes of SSVF that emerged as features to comprehensively deliver support for homeless veterans and their families: (1) responsiveness and flexibility, (2) coordination and integration, and (3) social resource engagement.

Using these strategies, SSVF reached nearly three quarters of a million veterans and their families in its first decade, thereby becoming one of the VA's most substantial programmatic efforts designed to address homelessness. We discuss how each feature might apply to addressing homelessness in the general population as well as future research directions. (*Am J Public Health*. 2024;114(6):610–618. https://doi.org/10.2105/AJPH.2024.307625)

AJPH June 2024, Vol. 114, No. 6

Although national rates of homelessness continue to increase,[1] the striking overall reduction among veterans over the past decade is a source of hope for policymakers, practitioners, researchers, and the public. Although the precise causes have not been determined, the decrease has followed more than a decade of the federal government's targeted efforts aimed specifically at eliminating veteran homelessness. We comprehensively review a program central to these efforts: Supportive Services for Veteran Families (SSVF).

The US Department of Veterans Affairs (VA) has addressed the problem of veteran homelessness for nearly 4 decades, beginning in 1987, when Congress passed the landmark Stewart B. McKinney Homeless Assistance Act.[2] This act established the Health Care for Homeless Veterans Program—the first federal program to specifically address the needs of veterans experiencing homelessness.[3] Five years later, investment expanded when the Homeless Veterans Comprehensive Services Act allowed the VA and the US Department of Housing and Urban Development (HUD) to collaboratively establish the HUD–VA Supportive Housing (HUD–VASH) program; this provides permanent supportive housing, and the Grant and Per Diem program, which provides transitional housing. Both became permanent VA programs in 2001.[4]

In 2007, estimates from the first Annual Homeless Assessment Report to Congress indicated that veterans (18.7%) remained overrepresented in the homeless shelter population compared with the general population (12.6%), a finding consistently reported in the following years.[5] This elevated risk stemmed from factors related to military service (e.g., combat exposure, posttraumatic stress disorder) and postmilitary life (e.g., job loss, relationship dissolution), as well as other complicating issues (e.g., substance use disorders, low income).[6,7] Such risk poses a threat to veterans' well-being because homelessness is linked to a wide array of adverse health outcomes, including an increased risk of mortality.[8]

The pressing needs of veterans returning from the wars in Iraq and Afghanistan prompted bipartisan efforts to reduce homelessness and improve support mechanisms.[9] In the early 2000s, no existing VA homeless program explicitly focused on preventing veteran homelessness, preventing veteran family homelessness, or providing direct financial assistance. In 2008, however, the Veterans' Mental Health and Other Care Improvements Act authorized the VA to create SSVF, a program that began in 2012 to prevent homelessness among at-risk veterans and their families or to rapidly rehouse them if they were already homeless. That same year, universal screening for housing instability was introduced for all veterans accessing VA outpatient services.

In 2009, the federal government, in announcing a national goal to eliminate veteran homelessness over the next decade, established the National Center on Homelessness Among Veterans through additional funding for HUD–VASH, the SSVF, and the Grant and Per Diem programs; the center was codified under the Veterans Health Care and Benefits Improvement Act of 2016.[10] From 2008 to 2022, veteran homelessness decreased by an estimated 46.8% (Table 1), which far exceeded the 4.9% reduction in homelessness among the nonveteran population during the same period. Veterans are no longer overrepresented among those experiencing homelessness. In 2022, the Biden administration introduced All In: The Federal Strategic Plan to Prevent and End Homelessness, which highlighted the remarkable reduction in veteran homelessness as a roadmap for addressing the crisis nationwide.[11]

Although several previous publications have analyzed specific SSVF features, such as type of housing assistance received[12] and temporary financial assistance provision,[13] to our knowledge, no study to date has comprehensively reviewed the program's overall features and operations. In consultation with key program administrators, we provide the first such review by analyzing all SSVF annual reports used to inform Congress and the public about program operations and outcomes as well as relevant literature published since the program's inception. This allowed us to identify 3 key themes from SSVF policies and practices that contributed to the goal of reducing veterans' homelessness: (1) flexibility and responsiveness, (2) coordination and integration, and (3)

TABLE 1— Point-in-Time Estimates for People Experiencing Homelessness: United States, 2008–2022

		Veterans		
Year	All People, No.	All Veterans, No. (% of All People)	Sheltered, No.	Unsheltered, No. (% of All Veterans)
2008	639 784	62 223 (9.73)	38 485	23 738 (38.15)
2009	630 227	73 367 (11.64)	43 409	29 958 (40.83)
2010	637 077	74 087 (11.63)	43 437	30 650 (41.37)
2011	623 788	65 455 (10.49)	40 033	25 422 (38.84)
2012	621 553	60 579 (9.75)	35 143	25 436 (41.99)
2013	590 364	55 619 (9.42)	34 909	20 710 (37.24)
2014	576 450	49 689 (8.62)	32 119	17 570 (35.36)
2015	564 708	47 725 (8.45)	31 505	16 220 (33.99)
2016	549 928	39 471 (7.18)	26 404	13 067 (33.11)
2017	550 996	40 020 (7.26)	24 690	15 330 (38.31)
2018	552 830	37 878 (6.85)	23 312	14 566 (38.46)
2019	567 715	37 085 (6.53)	22 740	14 345 (38.68)
2020	580 466	37 252 (6.42)	22 048	15 204 (40.81)
2021[a]	. . .	. . .	19 750	. . .
2022	582 462	33 129 (5.69)	19 565	13 564 (40.94)

Note. All point-in-time estimates reported in the table were sourced from the 2023 Annual Homeless Assessment Report.[1]
[a]Estimates for 2021 were omitted because of challenges conducting unsheltered point-in-time counts during the COVID-19 pandemic.

social resource engagement. Lessons learned from SSVF can inform broader national efforts focused on addressing the pressing issue of homelessness.

PROGRAM DESCRIPTION

Among VA homeless programs, SSVF is unique in its focus on veterans and their families. It aims either to rapidly rehouse those who are literally homeless (e.g., living in an emergency shelter or a place unintended for human habitation), with the goal of finding permanent housing, or to prevent homelessness for those at imminent risk for losing housing. SSVF provides grants to community-based nonprofit organizations ("grantees") to coordinate or provide supportive services to low-income veteran households; "low income," initially defined as below 50% of the area's median income, was redefined as up to 80% of area median income (as of fiscal year [FY] 2023) to align with HUD–VASH.

In its first year, SSVF provided $59.5 million to 85 grantees. Grants ranged from $41 000 to $1 000 000 and served approximately 21 100 veteran households, collectively benefiting more than 35 000 adults and children.[14] By 2021, expenditures increased to $633 million annually provided to 251 grantees, serving approximately 80 924 veteran households and collectively benefiting more than 116 000 adults and children.[15] New funding proposals in 2022 allowed each grantee to request a maximum of $4 million, with no more than $9000 of budgeted support per veteran household.[16]

Early iterations of SSVF were informed by the HUD federal Homelessness Prevention and Rapid Rehousing Program (HPRP), which was funded by the American Recovery and Reinvestment Act of 2009. This initiative, ending in 2012, worked with local governments and community-based organizations to address the most severe consequences of the Great Recession (2007–2009) on individuals and families with low incomes. HPRP focused mostly on prevention but was notable for its efforts to provide rapid rehousing, short-term financial services, and additional supportive resources.[17] SSVF did not simply replicate HPRP but rather built on lessons learned from it. For example, SSVF focused more on rehousing veterans who were literally experiencing homelessness (per the federal definition).[18] In fact, on average, 70% of SSVF participants who were literally experiencing homelessness at entry were served with rapid rehousing services (those imminently at risk for literal homelessness at entry received homelessness prevention assistance). Additionally, although HPRP allowed providers to develop their own eligibility criteria in the broad framework of HUD guidelines, SSVF created a standardized research-informed screening tool, which is integrated into HUD's Homeless Management Information System and is now completed by all SSVF grantees to assess risk and eligibility for prevention services.[19]

From 2012 to 2022, SSVF served more than 732 000 veterans and dependent family members, with a 79% rate of exit to permanent housing[15]; these efforts occurred against a backdrop of a 300% increase in rapid rehousing beds for the broader unhoused population nationwide between 2014 and 2022.[20] Notably, SSVF serves a wide array of participants. For example, in FY 2021, more than half (53%) identified as a Black, Indigenous, or other person of color.[8] SSVF also served the largest proportion of veteran women (13%) of any VA homeless initiative.[15] Approximately 70% of all veterans served by SSVF had extremely low incomes (area median income < 30%). Approximately, 18% of SSVF participants were dependent children.

SSVF differs from other VA homeless programs in a number of ways. First, it works exclusively through community organizations (unlike Domiciliary Care for Homeless Veterans, which is a residential program with a physical presence on VA grounds). Second, services are time limited and aim to assist veterans who do not require long-term supports (as opposed to HUD–VASH, which involves extended case management and usually enrolls veterans with disabling conditions). Third, it provides services, including childcare, to help keep families intact, which can continue for up to 1 year even after a veteran departs the program. Fourth, SSVF emphasizes rapid rehousing with supportive services as a means of achieving and maintaining permanent housing in the community.

Figure 1 illustrates the general SSVF process of entry, engagement, and exit. Candidates are first screened for eligibility (e.g., having < 80% area median income, experiencing homelessness or being imminently at risk for experiencing homelessness).[15] Individualized housing stability plans, devised for each enrollee, aim to facilitate obtaining permanent housing and subsequently exiting SSVF. Each participant's progress is monitored in the context of their housing stability plan, with modifications made based on changing needs. Participants exit SSVF when they are self-sufficient in sustaining housing.

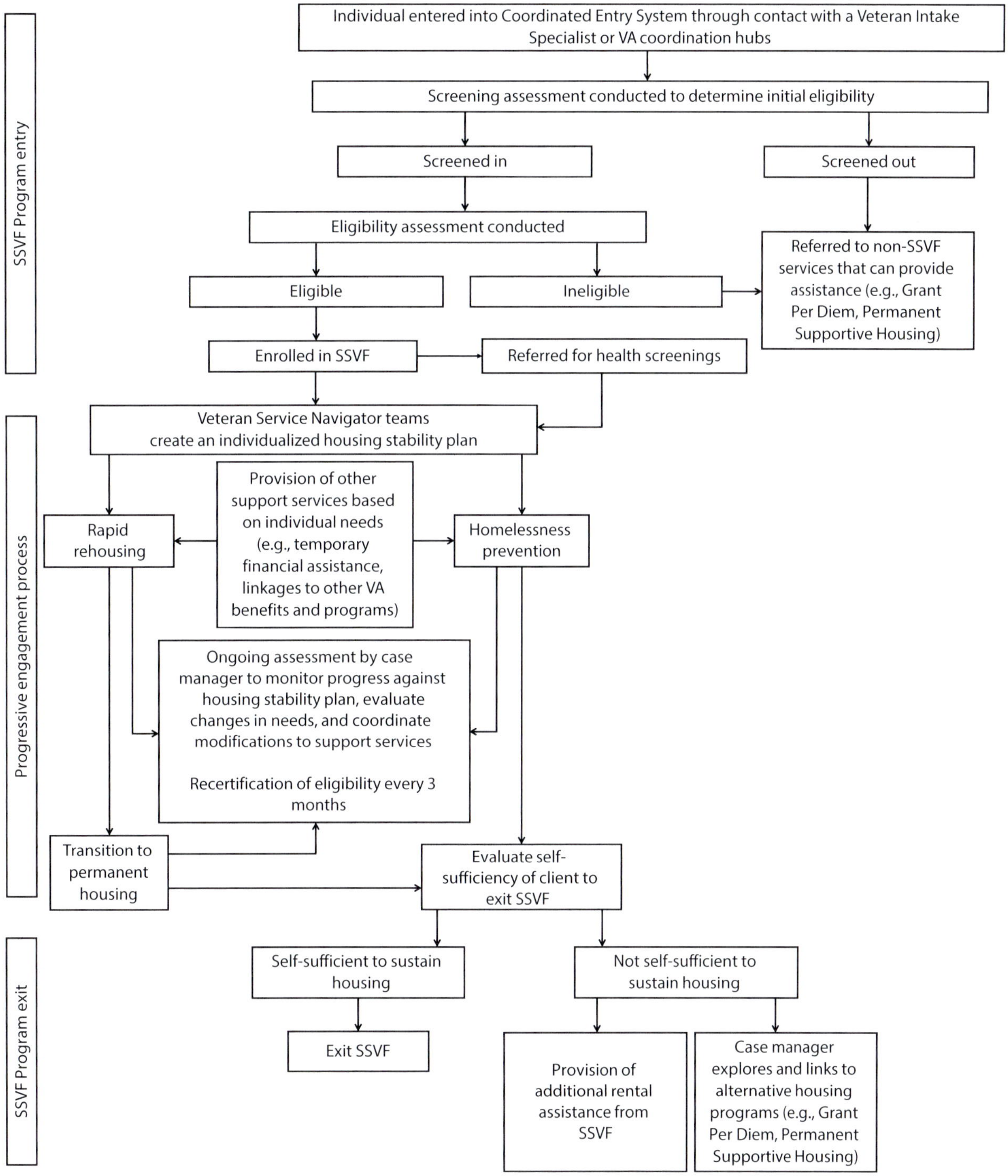

FIGURE 1— Flowchart of SSVF Program Entry, Engagement, and Exit

Note. SSVF = Supportive Services for Veteran Families; VA = Veterans Affairs.

IMPORTANT FIRST-DECADE THEMES

To further illustrate how SSVF operates and contributes to efforts to reduce veteran homelessness, we explored 3 program themes across its first decade of existence: (1) responsiveness and flexibility, (2) coordination and integration, and (3) social resource engagement.

Responsiveness and Flexibility

SSVF evolved to address both macro- and individual-level contributors to housing insecurity. Macrolevel events (e.g., natural disasters and economic downturns) can immediately threaten veterans' housing security and require timely and flexible response. For example, in the aftermath of the Great Recession, increasing demand for housing alongside decreasing supply of new housing units forced lower-income renters to compete for available rental housing. In the following decade, these pressures persisted in high-cost, low-vacancy communities. In 2022, the United States had a shortage of approximately 7.3 million affordable and available homes for renters with extremely low incomes, with only 33 homes available for every 100 households in need.[21]

In response, SSVF relies heavily on landlords accepting rental payments from grantees to house homeless veterans and their families. For example, in FY 2019, SSVF launched the Shallow Subsidy initiative in 11 pilot communities. The initiative provided additional rental support for up to 2 years, capped at 35% of the local HUD fair market rate. Veterans received a constant subsidy not subject to income recertification, which allowed them to increase their income during the 2-year period without risking loss of the housing subsidy and other benefits. Early data suggest that veterans who participated in the Shallow Subsidy initiative exited the program with higher levels of income; more evaluation of housing, economic, and health outcomes is currently under way.[22]

In 2021, SSVF expanded the Shallow Subsidy initiative by increasing both the number of participating states and the subsidy rate (to 50% of rent); it also changed the basis of the subsidy to "rent reasonableness" from fair market rate (which trails market rates). In its opening year, FY 2021, the Shallow Subsidy initiative served 1113 veterans in 24 US states (and Washington, DC), of whom 70% received rapid rehousing and 30% received prevention assistance.[15] SSVF also partnered with other federal agencies to coenroll veterans in employment and training programs aimed at improving their likelihood of economic self-sufficiency.[23] In FY 2022, the Shallow Subsidy initiative served more than 45 000 veterans across all 50 US states (and Washington, DC).

SSVF also demonstrated flexibility in response to natural disasters by using unspent grantee funds to support emergency relief efforts for veterans and their families.[24] Such flexibility became essential early in the COVID-19 pandemic, when SSVF directed VA medical centers to work with grantees to identify homeless veterans needing placement in hotels and motels as part of social-distancing measures. Such actions were among the earliest federal responses to address the unique risks faced by persons experiencing homelessness. Ultimately, SSVF placed more than 32 000 veteran households in hotels or motels between March 2020 and September 2021.[15] Recent evidence shows that these pandemic efforts served an especially vulnerable population of veterans, including those who were previously unsheltered or resistant to services.[25]

Moreover, the Stafford Act and the Coronavirus Aid, Relief, and Economic Security (CARES) Act of 2020 allowed SSVF to extend the time during the pandemic that veterans and their families could stay in temporary housing.[23] By increasing coordination with HUD–VASH in providing supportive housing and removing limits on the number of months of rental assistance, SSVF helped veterans and their families remain in stable housing during this time. Such flexibilities enabled SSVF to serve 55 018 veterans with rapid rehousing by the end of FY 2020, an increase of 3068 from FY 2019.[15] Despite staying in the system longer—which was potentially associated with higher program costs—many veterans in fact needed a lighter touch (i.e., limited intervention and support), and overall transition rates to permanent housing (> 70%) mirrored historic averages.[15,23]

SSVF's responsiveness and flexibility also helped grantees to overcome local-level challenges. For example, grantees in several communities, including rural and tribal areas, initially found it difficult to meet the SSVF requirement that at least 60% of expenditures support rapid rehousing services rather than prevention. In response, from FY 2016 to FY 2018, SSVF developed a waiver process allowing more flexibility for funds spent at the local level. From FY 2014 to FY 2017, 67 high-priority communities with large concentrations of homeless veterans received an additional $289 million to support higher program costs incurred

(SSVF annual budgets grew from $241 million in 2014 to $414 million in 2017).[26] SSVF also increased technical support, as exemplified by its Program Manager Academy, which offered short intensive training for new program managers to better navigate their local contexts.[23]

At the individual level, SSVF addressed the unique needs and circumstances of each veteran family. During the design phase of SSVF, the VA analyzed a long-standing survey on veteran homelessness[27] to identify family needs, resulting in an early emphasis on family services such as childcare, access to legal services, and additional financial support for victims of domestic violence.[28] In another example, because grantees initially reported having to turn away eligible families owing to limits on the use of financial assistance, in FY 2013, SSVF increased the limit on temporary financial assistance from 30% to 50% of supportive services grant funding.[28] Additionally, the Rapid Resolution initiative, piloted in FY 2018 and expanded nationwide in FY 2020, helped veterans experiencing a housing crisis identify alternatives to emergency shelters or the streets by using unique social support networks of individual veterans (e.g., housing with extended family or friends).[29]

Coordination and Integration

SSVF has long operated with extensive coordination and integration with other programs and initiatives, both inside and outside the VA. In 2014, the SSVF Program Office began tracking grantee and community partner progress toward effectively ending homelessness among veterans. Such tracking efforts, first initiated in 71 priority communities, expanded in 2015 to include all grantees and the communities served.[26] In addition, in 2016, it began working closely with the US Interagency Council on Homelessness and HUD to assess and identify local needs, develop coordinated technical assistance, and implement evidence-based strategies. Such efforts helped all parties better assess community efforts regarding functional leadership, plans with actionable strategies, and practices that align with federal efforts.

Because the COVID-19 pandemic complicated access to services, SSVF provided dedicated support to connect program participants with health resources. One opportunity in 2020 allowed SSVF to award $400 million in supplemental funding (through the CARES Act) for grantees to employ health care navigators, who coordinated care efforts between VA medical centers and other health care systems.[23]

As part of this, SSVF committed to coordination and continuity across VA services by providing resources to support grantees' local efforts through a common set of strategies and approaches for technical assistance, planning, and implementation.[23] Then, when public housing authorities suspended operations during the pandemic, many SSVF grantees increased support for veterans eligible for both SSVF and HUD–VASH to allow time to coordinate receiving available vouchers and units. A community of practice sessions that connected grantees to local HUD–VASH facilitated this process.[23]

Moreover, SSVF coordinated with the Grant and Per Diem program to provide "bridge" housing that addressed a veteran's immediate need for safety and shelter, reduced the need for time-consuming street outreach while leases were formalized, and ensured direct, rapid access to permanent housing.[15] SSVF grantees also helped veterans gain permanent housing through HUD–VASH and employment assistance through the Department of Labor's Homeless Veterans' Reintegration Program.[15] These collective approaches likely conserved resources and minimized duplication of services funded by other VA programs (Figure 1).

SSVF also facilitated integration with other federal agencies to increase income and health care support that allowed sustained permanent housing. Through the Supplemental Security Income (SSI) and Social Security Disability Insurance (SSDI) Outreach, Access, and Recovery Initiative, for example, SSVF helped veterans obtain or retain stable housing by providing a consistent, sizable income source and health care access for veterans at risk for homelessness with a mental illness, medical impairment, or cooccurring substance use disorder.[26] This program, funded by the Substance Abuse and Mental Health Services Administration, helped eligible veterans overcome barriers—including lack of medical, employment, and educational history—to obtain SSI/SSDI benefits. Recent data from the SSI/SSDI Outreach, Access, and Recovery Initiative program demonstrate its impact. For example, in 2021, persons experiencing homelessness who received SSI/SSDI Outreach, Access, and Recovery Initiative assistance had their disability determination approved at a rate of 60% to 65% (vs an average rate of 10%–15% without such assistance between 2006 and 2021).[30]

SSVF also connects veterans with community-based organizations to support long-term housing stability and general welfare. Such organizations provide training programs, employment support, food assistance programs, mental health and substance use programs, childcare assistance, and Temporary Assistance for Needy Families benefits. Integrating SSVF services with these additional forms of assistance increases the efficient use of resources, facilitates continuity of support, addresses underlying factors contributing to housing instability and homelessness, and connects veterans and their families with organizations that can provide long-term support.

Social Resource Engagement

SSVF's emphasis on keeping families together has particular importance for women veterans, who are often the caregivers of dependent children. FY 2018 data showed that among SSVF households with children that included a woman veteran, 73% had no other adult in the household and no (or only partial) child support.[29] Notably, SSVF provides support for up to a year for a veteran and their family, even after they no longer live together. This allows SSVF to support family housing stability, especially for the children who constitute 20% of SSVF's participants. Additionally, in cases of separation owing to domestic violence, SSVF can rehouse the victim (even if they are a nonveteran) and provide the full range of services for up to 1 year.

Beginning in 2017, SSVF deployed 2 strategies to help veterans gain housing stability by reuniting them with their social networks. The Returning Home program recognized that 15% to 20% of homeless veterans migrated across the nation's 18 regional VA service networks,[29] often involving travel across high-cost, low-vacancy metropolitan areas without family and friends to provide vital support networks. Returning Home, piloted in 2017, provided veterans the option of returning to their communities of origin or to communities where they had such available support. It was then incorporated into the 2019 rollout of the Rapid Resolution initiative,[24] which aimed to reconnect veterans to family, friends, and others willing to provide a temporary or permanent residence.

As part of the initiative, SSVF grantees support family reunification through conflict resolution, de-escalation, motivational interviewing, and rapport building. It also offered targeted financial assistance for family or friends willing to house a veteran who lack financial resources to absorb associated costs. The Rapid Resolution initiative also helps veterans and their households access additional resources through employment and other appropriate benefits, thereby conserving deeper financial assistance packages for veterans who lack alternative pathways to permanent housing.

IMPLICATIONS FOR ADDRESSING HOMELESSNESS

Some features of SSVF can guide programs or policies that address homelessness in the general population, especially since it critically offers a "both/and" approach by focusing on individual and structural solutions. The literature has robustly documented that both structural factors (e.g., income inequality, tight rental markets)[31,32] and individual vulnerabilities (e.g., family structure, job loss)[33] can contribute to homelessness risk.[34]

SSVF grantees are empowered to use various resources available to craft unique solutions to address individual situations and goals. Such strategies, exemplified in SSVF's Shallow Subsidy initiative, can inform current local, state, or federal programs to provide rental subsidies building individual income capability, which may, in turn, promote longer-term financial housing stability. In fact, other nonfederal efforts at the state, county, and city levels are initiating their own "shallow subsidy" financial assistance pilot programs to help low-income and at-risk individuals in the general population gain housing and financial stability. For example, California is currently pursuing a pilot program to provide shallow rental subsidies for older adults and disabled individuals.[35] Relatedly, in 2022, Chicago and Cook County, Illinois, launched guaranteed income pilots (using American Rescue Plan Act funding) to provide unconditional cash assistance of $500 per month to residents, particularly those experiencing economic hardship following the COVID-19 pandemic.[36]

Formal evaluations of these programs—along with the aforementioned ongoing study of SSVF's Shallow Subsidy initiative—will help researchers and policymakers understand the impact of different types of subsidies that address housing instability specifically (e.g., rental subsidies) and economic challenges more broadly (e.g., guaranteed income stipends), as well as the costs associated with these forms of support.

SSVF's approach of fostering and deepening organizational relationships across a wide spectrum can also inform programs for the general population. By collaborating with both federal agencies and community organizations to jointly meet the needs of veterans and their families, SSVF can efficiently use resources, facilitate continuity of support, and address underlying factors associated with housing instability and homelessness, which often require multiple-party support. Homelessness programs targeting the general population can draw on VA practices by deepening and expanding multisectoral partnership networks into a multilayered collection of services and resources. Enhanced dialogue between the VA and other national groups may lead to opportunities to exchange knowledge and share resources (e.g., best practices, screening tools) to enhance services for those in need. It can also improve the way researchers and policymakers evaluate what works best in organizations and communities.

SSVF's recognition that social relationships play an essential role in the lives of veterans who experience homelessness might also foster broader national efforts. Such an "asset-based approach" can reconnect veterans with their social networks and restore relationships with friends and family, which may in turn bolster community connections, promote belonging, address loneliness and stigma, and ultimately advance well-being.[37] Although some individuals experiencing homelessness have histories of unhealthy relationships, there may be members in their social network who can help, if given sufficient support.[38]

LIMITATIONS AND FUTURE DIRECTIONS

We have provided the first, to our knowledge, comprehensive overview of SSVF and the ways it may have contributed to addressing veteran homelessness over the past decade. We distilled our descriptive analysis principally from SSVF annual reports, discussions with VA's Homeless Programs Office, and internal literature. Hence, additional rigorous research and a more formal evaluation are needed to formally assess the impact of SSVF and its various components on veteran housing, health, and social outcomes.

Notably, the diverse modes of SSVF implementation and variety of needs served make it challenging to make comparisons with other large-scale social programs. Encouragingly, however, an emerging body of such research includes several studies examining specific components of SSVF; receipt of temporary financial assistance, for example, has been associated with increased likelihood of program exit to stable housing[12,39] and lower health care costs.[40]

Ongoing studies will provide future evidence about the effects of the Shallow Subsidy initiative as well as the overall impact of the rapid rehousing component of SSVF on various outcomes.[21] Additional research could explore whether site-to-site differences in SSVF implementation are related to site-to-site differences in outcomes, as well as the generalizability of applying the SSVF model to other populations.

CONCLUSIONS

Examining and learning from complex, flexible, and tailored programs like SSVF can inform the general medical and public health community and serve as a foundation for other innovative programs. Three key features of SSVF—(1) flexibility and responsiveness, (2) coordination and integration, and (3) social resource engagement—appear to have contributed to SSVF's operational success during its first decade, including the program's evolution in response to the social and economic challenges of the pandemic. Such factors have enabled SSVF to serve nearly 750 000 veterans and their families. Alongside other VA programs and federal resources dedicated to preventing and reducing veteran homelessness, the cornerstone program of SSVF may hold promise for application to addressing the crisis in the general population. AJPH

ABOUT THE AUTHORS

Renae Wilkinson, Richard G. Cowden, and Katelyn N. G. Long are with the Human Flourishing Program, Institute for Quantitative Social Science, Harvard University, Cambridge, MA. Thomas Byrne is with the School of Social Work, Boston University, Boston, MA. John H. Kuhn is with the VA Greater Los Angeles Healthcare System, Los Angeles, CA. Howard K. Koh is with the Harvard T. H. Chan School of Public Health, Boston, MA. Jack Tsai is with the US Department of Veterans Affairs, National Center on Homelessness Among Veterans, Washington DC.

CORRESPONDENCE

Correspondence should be sent to Jack Tsai, PhD, MSCP, 1200 Pressler St, Houston, TX 77030 (e-mail: Jack.Tsai@uth.tmc.edu). Reprints can be ordered at http://www.ajph.org by clicking the "Reprints" link.

PUBLICATION INFORMATION

Full Citation: Wilkinson R, Byrne T, Cowden RG, et al. First decade of Supportive Services for Veteran Families Program and homelessness, 2012–2022. *Am J Public Health*. 2024;114(6): 610–618.

Acceptance Date: February 8, 2024.

DOI: https://doi.org/10.2105/AJPH.2024.307625

CONTRIBUTORS

R. Wilkinson, R. G. Cowden, and K. N. G. Long conceptualized, conducted research for, and wrote the essay. T. Byrne, H. K. Koh, J. H. Kuhn, and J. Tsai contributed to writing and revisions. All authors approved the final version to be published.

ACKNOWLEDGMENTS

Funding was provided in part by the US Department of Veterans Affairs and the Harvard T. H. Chan Initiative on Health and Homelessness.

We give special thanks to Marian M. Jones for her comments on the essay draft and to Tyler J. VanderWeele, PhD, for his support of this work.

CONFLICTS OF INTEREST

The authors have no conflicts of interest to declare.

HUMAN PARTICIPANT PROTECTION

Institutional review board approval was not needed for this work because there were no human participants involved.

REFERENCES

1. US Department of Housing and Urban Development. The 2023 annual homeless assessment report (AHAR) to Congress. 2023. Available at: https://www.huduser.gov/portal/sites/default/files/pdf/2023-AHAR-Part-1.pdf. Accessed December 20, 2023.
2. Gabbard WJ, Ford B, May JD. The Stewart B. McKinney Homeless Assistance Act: a historical overview. *J Soc Distress Homeless.* 2006;15(2):99–115. https://doi.org/10.1179/sdh.2006.15.2.99
3. Perl L. Veterans and homelessness. April 12, 2023. CRS report no. RL34024. Available at: https://sgp.fas.org/crs/misc/RL34024.pdf. Accessed March 23, 2024.
4. Tsai J, O'Connell M, Kasprow WJ, Rosenheck RA. Factors related to rapidity of housing placement in Housing and Urban Development–Department of Veterans Affairs Supportive Housing Program of 1990s. *J Rehabil Res Dev.* 2011;48(7):755–762. https://doi.org/10.1682/JRRD.2010.09.0178
5. US Department of Housing and Urban Development. The annual homeless assessment report to Congress. February 2007. Available at: https://www.huduser.gov/portal/sites/default/files/pdf/ahar.pdf. Accessed December 2, 2023.
6. Metraux S, Clegg LX, Daigh JD, Culhane DP, Kane V. Risk factors for becoming homeless among a cohort of veterans who served in the era of the Iraq and Afghanistan conflicts. *Am J Public Health.* 2013;103(suppl 2):S255–S261. https://doi.org/10.2105/AJPH.2013.301432
7. Tsai J, Rosenheck RA. Risk factors for homelessness among US veterans. *Epidemiol Rev.* 2015;37:177–195. https://doi.org/10.1093/epirev/mxu004
8. Fazel S, Geddes JR, Kushel M. The health of homeless people in high-income countries: descriptive epidemiology, health consequences, and clinical and policy recommendations. *Lancet.* 2014;384(9953):1529–1540. https://doi.org/10.1016/S0140-6736(14)61132-6
9. Tsai J. *Homelessness Among US Veterans: Critical Perspectives.* New York, NY: Oxford University Press; 2019.
10. US Interagency Council on Homelessness. *Opening Doors: Federal Strategic Plan to Prevent and End Homelessness.* Washington, DC; 2010.
11. US Interagency Council on Homelessness. *All In: The Federal Strategic Plan to Prevent and End Homelessness.* Washington, DC; 2022.
12. Byrne T, Montgomery AE, Chapman AB, et al. Predictors of homeless service utilization and stable housing status among veterans receiving services from a nationwide homelessness prevention and rapid rehousing program. *Eval Program Plann.* 2023;97:102223. https://doi.org/10.1016/j.evalprogplan.2022.102223
13. Nelson RE, Byrne T, Zickmund SL, et al. Which veterans in the Supportive Services for Veteran Families Program receive temporary financial assistance and why: a mixed methods study. *J Soc Distress Homeless.* 2023;32:210–222. https://doi.org/10.1080/10530789.2022.2035147
14. US Department of Veterans Affairs. *Supportive Services for Veteran Families (SSVF) FY 2012 Annual Report.* Washington, DC; 2012.
15. US Department of Veterans Affairs. *FY 2021 Annual Report: Supportive Services for Veteran Families.* Washington, DC: Supportive Services for Veteran Families; 2021.
16. Martin JM. Funding opportunity under Supportive Services for Veteran Families Program. *Fed Regist.* 2022;87(207):65119–65126.
17. US Department of Housing and Urban Development. Homelessness Prevention and Rapid Rehousing Program (HPRP): year 3 & final program summary. 2016. Available at: https://files.hudexchange.info/resources/documents/HPRP-Year-3-Summary.pdf. Accessed March 22, 2024.
18. US Department of Housing and Urban Development. Four categories of the homeless definition. Available at: https://www.hudexchange.info/homelessness-assistance/coc-esg-virtual-binders/coc-esg-homeless-eligibility/four-categories. Accessed December 1, 2023.
19. US Department of Veterans Affairs. Supportive Services for Veteran Families (SSVF) homelessness prevention screening tool companion guide. September 2021. Available at: https://www.va.gov/HOMELESS/ssvf/docs/SSVF_HP_Screening_Companion_Guide.pdf. Accessed December 29, 2023.
20. de Sousa T, Andrichik A, Cuellar M, Marson J, Prestera E, Rush K. The 2022 annual homelessness assessment report (AHAR) to Congress. December 2022. Available at: https://www.huduser.gov/portal/sites/default/files/pdf/2022-ahar-part-1.pdf. Accessed March 23, 2024.
21. National Low Income Housing Coalition. The GAP report: a shortage of affordable rental homes. 2023. Available at: https://nlihc.org/sites/default/files/gap/Gap-Report_2023.pdf. Accessed March 23, 2024.
22. US Department of Veterans Affairs. Health services research & development SDR 20-350 assessing an initiative to facilitate long-term financial and housing stability in vulnerable veterans. Available at: https://www.hsrd.research.va.gov/research/abstracts.cfm?Project_ID=2141709162. Accessed December 15, 2023.
23. US Department of Veterans Affairs. *FY 2020 Annual Report: Supportive Services for Veteran Families.* 2020. Available at: https://www.va.gov/HOMELESS/ssvf/docs/SSVF_Annual_Report_FY20.pdf. Accessed March 23, 2024.
24. US Department of Veterans Affairs. *FY 2019 Annual Report: Supportive Services for Veteran Families.* 2019. Available at: https://www.va.gov/homeless/ssvf/docs/SSVF_Annual_Report_FY19.pdf. Accessed March 23, 2024.
25. Montgomery AE, Zickmund S, Byrne TH, et al. The use of hotels/motels to address homelessness among veterans during the COVID-19 pandemic: lessons from the Supportive Services for Veteran Families Program. *J Soc Distress Homeless.* [Published online: March 10, 2023]. https://doi.org/10.1080/10530789.2023.2187522
26. US Department of Veterans Affairs. Supportive Services for Veteran Families (SSVF) FY 2015 annual report. 2015. Available at: https://www.va.gov/HOMELESS/ssvf/docs/SSVF_Annual_Report_FY15.pdf. Accessed March 23, 2024.
27. Tsai J, Blue-Howells J, Nakashima J. Needs of homeless veterans: 5 years of the CHALENG survey 2012–16. *J Public Health (Oxf).* 2019;41(1):e16–e24. https://doi.org/10.1093/pubmed/fdy076
28. US Department of Veterans Affairs. Supportive Services for Veteran Families (SSVR) FY 2013 annual report. 2013. Available at: https://www.va.gov/HOMELESS/ssvf/docs/SSVF_Annual_Report_FY13.pdf. Accessed March 23, 2024.
29. US Department of Veterans Affairs. FY 2018 annual report: Supportive Services for Veteran Families. 2019. Available at: https://www.va.gov/homeless/ssvf/docs/SSVF_FY2018_AnnualReport_508.pdf. Accessed March 23, 2024.
30. Substance Abuse and Mental Health Services Administration. National outcomes 2021. Available at: https://soarworks.samhsa.gov/sites/default/files/article/upload-files/2022-10/2021OutcomesInfographic.pdf. Accessed June 1, 2023.
31. Byrne T, Munley EA, Fargo JD, Montgomery AE, Culhane DP. New perspectives on community-level determinants of homelessness. *J Urban Aff.* 2013;35(5):607–625. https://doi.org/10.1111/j.1467-9906.2012.00643.x
32. Hanratty M. Do local economic conditions affect homelessness? Impact of area housing market factors, unemployment, and poverty on community homeless rates. *Hous Policy Debate.* 2017;27(4):640–655. https://doi.org/10.1080/10511482.2017.1282885
33. Giano Z, Williams A, Hankey C, Merrill R, Lisnic R, Herring A. Forty years of research on predictors of homelessness. *Community Ment Health J.* 2020;56(4):692–709. https://doi.org/10.1007/s10597-019-00530-5
34. Shinn M, Khadduri J. *In the Midst of Plenty: Homelessness and What to Do About It.* Hoboken, NJ: Wiley-Blackwell; 2020. https://doi.org/10.1002/9781119104780
35. Older Adults and Adults With Disabilities Housing Stability Act. California SB-37. Available at: https://trackbill.com/bill/california-senate-bill-37-older-adults-and-adults-with-disabilities-housing-stability-act/2282377. Accessed March 23, 2024.
36. City of Chicago Department of Family and Support Services. Chicago Resilient Communities pilot. Available at: https://www.chicago.gov/city/en/sites/resilient-communities-pilot/home.html. Accessed August 14, 2023.
37. Tate A, Edwards K, Holmes N, et al. "Even a smile helps": exploring the interactions between people experiencing homelessness and passersby in public spaces. *Int J Soc Psychiatry.* 2022;68(3):525–532. https://doi.org/10.1177/0020764021989385
38. O'Connell MJ, Rosenheck R. The family ties that bind: tangible, instrumental, and emotional support among homeless veterans. In: MacDermid Wadsworth S, Riggs D, eds. *War and Family Life. Risk and Resilience in Military and Veteran Families.* Cham, Germany: Springer; 2016. https://doi.org/10.1007/978-3-319-21488-7_15
39. Nelson RE, Byrne TH, Suo Y, et al. Association of temporary financial assistance with housing stability among US veterans in the Supportive Services for Veteran Families program. *JAMA Netw Open.* 2021;4(2):e2037047. https://doi.org/10.1001/jamanetworkopen.2020.37047
40. Nelson RE, Montgomery AE, Suo Y, et al. Temporary financial assistance decreased health care costs for veterans experiencing housing instability. *Health Aff (Millwood).* 2021;40(5):820–828. https://doi.org/10.1377/hlthaff.2020.01796

Building the Infrastructure to Integrate Social Care in a Safety Net Health System

Christopher M. Callahan, MD, Amy Carter, MA, RDN, Hannah S. Carty, MSPH, Daniel O. Clark, PhD, Tedd Grain, MPA, MA, Seth L. Grant, CDM, CFPP, Kimberly McElroy-Jones, PhD, Deanna Reinoso, MD, and Lisa E. Harris, MD

See also Silberberg, p. 543.

A recent National Academies report recommended that health systems invest in new infrastructure to integrate social and medical care. Although many health systems routinely screen patients for social concerns, few health systems achieve the recommended model of integration.

In this critical case study in an urban safety net health system, we describe the human capital, operational redesign, and financial investment needed to implement the National Academy recommendations. Using data from this case study, we estimate that other health systems seeking to build and maintain this infrastructure would need to invest $1 million to $3 million per year.

While health systems with robust existing resources may be able to bootstrap short-term funding to initiate this work, we conclude that long-term investments by insurers and other payers will be necessary for most health systems to achieve the recommended integration of medical and social care. Researchers seeking to test whether integrating social and medical care leads to better patient and population outcomes require access to health systems and communities who have already invested in this model infrastructure. (*Am J Public Health*. 2024;114(6):619–625. https://doi.org/10.2105/AJPH.2024.307602)

AJPH June 2024, Vol. 114, No. 6

The National Academies of Science, Engineering, and Medicine (NASEM) concluded that social care must be better integrated into the delivery of health care.[1] Previous NASEM reports, as well as the World Health Organization, concluded that social determinants of health and related social care issues contribute directly to health disparities and preventable chronic conditions.[2–6] The 2019 NASEM report suggested that to improve individual and population health, health systems must attend to social care as well as medical care. To realize these improvements in health, the NASEM report recommended substantive investments in the health care infrastructure including "the redesign and refinement of workflows, technical assistance and support, staff with the ability to support the redesign, champions of the redesign, information on best practices, health information technology to enhance integration, and support for community partners and their infrastructure needs."[1(p11)]

The goal of this essay is to describe a critical case study of a safety net health system seeking to build and sustain this recommended infrastructure without support from third-party payers. Although many federal agencies advocate for health systems to attend to social factors, third-party payers do not reimburse health systems for investments in the infrastructure to support this integration,[1,7] and potential cost savings do not necessarily accrue to the health system supporting the investment. Although many health systems already report efforts to routinely screen and refer patients to community resources, we are not aware of previous studies reporting on the resources and costs of health system redesign at the level of complexity recommended by the NASEM report.

In one of the larger demonstration projects to date, Lindau et al. used health information technology to enhance integration and provide technical support to staff.[8] Funded by the Center for Medicare and Medicaid Innovation, the team reported the outcomes of CommunityRx: "a scalable, low-intensity intervention that matches patients to community resources."[8(p600)] Not only did CommunityRx, a list of available resources generated through data in the electronic health record, increase patients' confidence in accessing community resources, but the patients also shared the resource information with others. An independent analysis of CommunityRx showed that the intervention was associated with a decrease in hospitalizations and an increase in primary care visits, but the study was not designed to determine if patients actually connected with the community service agency.[9] In a summary analysis of the Center for Medicare and Medicaid Innovation Accountable Health Communities, the authors found no significant increase in the rate of community service connections among patients with social needs referred to these service agencies.[10] Thus, the extant literature shows the potential of connecting patients reporting social needs with available services but also demonstrates that a more robust infrastructure may be needed to actually resolve the social needs. Here, we report on the challenges and costs of implementing the full palette of NASEM recommendations in a safety net health system serving a patient population burdened with both medical and social needs.

METHODS

We used the framework of a critical case analysis because the targeted health system offers unique opportunities to field test implementation of the new social care infrastructure.[11,12] We recognize that the setting is unique in some respects but also that our lessons learned may generalize to other settings. While we used the framework of a critical case study, some methodological frameworks might denote this approach as an extreme case, a positive deviance case, or an instrumental case study.[11,12] For example, from a financial perspective, this is a low-resource setting, outside the context of a research study, without substantive support from third-party payers for social care, and in service to a large population of urban-dwelling patients with a high prevalence of medical and social care needs. However, from a system's strength perspective, this safety net health system benefits from a strong existing neighborhood-based infrastructure, culture, and local community assets and trust. The challenges and lessons learned in this critical case study may offer the opportunity to instruct other health care systems who may be earlier in their evolution toward integrating social care and medical care. We report cost data using actual expenditures recorded in the health system's financial databases, which includes costs incurred by the health system but supported by philanthropic resources.

Eskenazi Health is the safety net health system serving Marion County, Indiana, which includes the city of Indianapolis. This health system meets the NASEM definition as Indianapolis' core safety net health system.[13] Among patients cared for over the past 5 years at Eskenazi Health, 41.3% identified as White, 33.4% as Black or African American, 1.9% as more than 1 race, and 1.4% as Asian (all other racial groups < 1%). In this same population, 12.5% self-identified their ethnicity as Hispanic. Among all patients, 11% preferred communication in Spanish, and 2% preferred to communicate in languages other than English or Spanish. Payor mix included Medicaid (45%), Medicare (28%), self-pay or uninsured (11%), and commercial (14%).

Eskenazi Health engenders a high level of trust in the local community and is recognized as the leading health system in Central Indiana for providing community benefit.[14] This health system includes a network of 14 neighborhood-based primary care centers (designated as a federally qualified health center) and 5 community mental health centers (a certified community behavioral health clinic). Each of these neighborhood-based centers is served by the same enterprise electronic health record (EHR) as the health system's inpatient and specialty services (Epic).

Eskenazi Health and the Marion County Public Health Department are divisions of the Health and Hospital Corporation of Marion County. These divisions collaborate on multiple efforts to improve the health of Indianapolis. This partnership includes colocation of medical care and public health services in the neighborhood-based clinics as well as collaboration in community outreach (e.g., vaccination), policy development (e.g., needle exchange), education (e.g., antiracism), and building the infrastructure to address the social determinants of health, including food insecurity, transportation, housing, and mental wellness. Thus, in these neighborhood-based clinics, we have colocation of primary care, behavioral health, and public health professionals.

RESULTS

Table 1 summarizes expenditures across all 6 NASEM-recommended infrastructure components.

TABLE 1— Annual Expenditures of Key NASEM-Recommended Health Care Infrastructure Components: 2019–2021

Infrastructure Component	Intramural Funds, $	Extramural Funds, Including Philanthropy, $
Champions of the redesign	629 000	111 000
Redesign of workflows	90 000	0
Health information technology	132 000	48 000
Technical and support staff	0	1 000 000
Community partners and their infrastructure needs	0	200 000
Information on best practices	100 000	50 000
Total	951 000	1 409 000

Note. NASEM = National Academies of Science, Engineering, and Medicine.

Champions of the Redesign

In 2018, Eskenazi Health leadership began the process to build a systemwide infrastructure to integrate medical care and social care, including direct financial support for a new team of leaders. We constructed this team to include a balance of expertise in the care of individuals and whole communities. The expertise in community-based care required external recruitment of champions with experience in community partnerships, neighborhood redevelopment, and economic development. This "champions of redesign" team was recruited over 3 years and now includes 7 leaders contributing a total of 3.8 full-time equivalents of effort. We value the current financial support for this leadership team at $740 000 per year. Philanthropy funded 15%, and the health system supported 85% of these costs over the past 3 years.

Redesign and Refinement of Workflows

Over the past half century, primary care successfully integrated multiple new activities into the workflow of the typical office visit. In addition to examples such as screening and treatment of hyperlipidemia, other activities integrated in the past few decades include counseling for smoking cessation, weight gain prevention, and other age-specific preventive health services. The basic workflow to integrate social care into health care includes familiar components: screening to identify individuals with problems followed by the options of counseling, treatment, or referral to address the problem, and then follow-up care to assure the problem is addressed.

However, 4 realities render the social care workflow more complex. First, there are no pharmaceutical or procedural options to assist in treatment of any of the social determinants of health. Second, social care interventions are not reimbursed by insurers. Third, most of the available services and supports to address social care problems reside outside of the health care system. Fourth, although this is a growing area of research, we need higher-quality studies supporting the scalability and sustainability of social care programming, including demonstrating improvements in patient-level outcomes or total health care costs.[15–17]

Community-based primary care is a logical service on which to integrate social care and medical care, if we provide appropriate additional resources in this setting. Our new care workflow relies on the workflow paradigm of screening, treatment or referral, and follow-up. This workflow also relies on a team-based care model already existing in our network of neighborhood-based health centers. Concurrent with investments in social care, Eskenazi Health invested $90 000 per year in consultant fees to work with our leadership and staff to build team-based approaches into the delivery of high-quality, efficient, patient-centric primary care. These new approaches address the responsibility and accountability of individual team members within the highly dynamic environment of primary care. Thus, integration of the social care role into the workflow of the expanding health care team represents a major infrastructure and cultural challenge.

Health Information Technology

Since 2018, the EHR at Eskenazi Health has supported screening for social determinants of health, and this information is displayed to providers like other health care data or reminders. Screening data can be collected by providers in clinic or by patients through the patient portal. The EHR also supports referral to a limited number of internal services such as financial counseling or assistance with application for the Supplemental Nutrition

Assistance Program. Although Eskenazi Health invests substantially in the EHR, this enterprise system (like many others) includes the main features needed to support screening and internal referral, so we do not attribute any financial investment in this key infrastructure directly to social care integration. The EHR can also provide written instruction for accessing a web-based directory of external community-based resources (https://www.findhelp.org). Accessing this directory and integrating it with the EHR in a format useable by patients and providers requires an average investment of $80 000 per year, which has been supported by philanthropy (60%) and the health system (40%) for the past 3 years.

The EHR does not capture data on whether a patient accessed services external to the health care system or the outcome of those services. Collecting such data requires follow-up communication with the patient or their advocates. Our inability to electronically "close the loop" between the health system and the community-based resources represents a major gap in the "screening–treatment–follow-up" paradigm. Although social network software can assist in finding resources, and to a limited extent can provide the technical capabilities to report back if a referral was completed, the process of closing the loop to better understand if services were requested by the patient and if they resolved their issue(s) remains underdeveloped for myriad technical, cultural, and regulatory reasons. We view these social network platforms as important tools but likely not sufficient alone to improve patient outcomes or health care costs.

As noted, the incremental cost of health information technology to support the screening components for social care is minimal, but the cost of building the workflow to address appropriate referral and follow-up is substantial. We value this EHR information technology support at a cost of $100 000 per year based on the hours of required programming and the cost per hour of the personnel to complete the programming. To date, this cost is borne primarily by the health system, and closing the communication gap with external resources is an important future step in innovation that could add substantially to costs.

Technical Assistance and Support Staff

The sum weight of all current recommended preventive care and chronic care management activities cannot be accomplished in a single ambulatory care visit by a single provider.[18,19] As noted, team-based care is now the norm within the framework of the neighborhood-based clinical practices. However, the composition of this team continues to evolve. We seek innovation in the composition of these teams to offset the new demands of integrating social care. Where a team might have consisted of a physician, nurse, social worker, and medical assistant over the past 10 years, this team now includes mental health social workers, registered dieticians, health coaches, community health workers, doulas, peer counselors, navigators, and financial counselors, among others, depending on the clinical site. While these new team members represent a welcomed new workforce, third-party payments fail to underwrite the full costs of this labor. In addition, these new roles require new enhancements in clinical communication and local adaptations based on local needs to assign roles, responsibilities, and accountability. We also identified an early need for a new role to help primary care patients navigate the ecosystem of community-based services. "Community weavers" identify resources in the neighborhoods surrounding each of our clinical sites, develop relationships with the leadership of these resources, and help patients navigate access. These 20 positions are funded through a combination of federal support to the primary care centers and local philanthropy.

Support for Community Partners

In the modal "screening–treatment–follow-up" medical paradigm, the entire process occurs under the umbrella of the health care organization. Although fragmentation and miscommunication continue to trouble this medical system, EHRs support communication about the outcomes of intramural referrals. When the referral process expands to include community-based organizations, we enter a much more complicated and heterogeneous network of services with unaligned technology and expectations. This heterogeneity stems from differences in what services are available in any given locality because of variation in the size, longevity, and administrative capacities of the organization. The range of information technology capabilities represents 1 example of this heterogeneity. Some highly valuable local organizations do not use software programs or, when available, such programs may be beyond the training available to their volunteer workforces. In some situations, the community-based organization, the client, or the health care system may be unwilling to allow sharing of information. For some larger organizations, such as Area Administrations on Aging, Eskenazi Health achieves a bidirectional flow of information, but these singular successes rarely generalize to other organizations.

Health care systems such as Eskenazi Health play an important role as anchor institutions in the neighborhoods where they provide services.[20] In this role, the health system provides employment and capital investment opportunities for local communities and offers administrative support for other activities, such as collaborative grant applications. Eskenazi Health offers the potential to expand administrative capacity in these organizations, but partnership also offers the potential to expand service capacity in these organizations. Patient needs exposed by widespread screening conducted by health systems easily overwhelm many community-based organizations.

As an example of a role for an anchor institution, Eskenazi Health partners with community-based organizations to achieve economies of scale for activities such as food service logistics, training and related workforce development, and neighborhood redevelopment. For these partnerships to be successful long-term, many community-based organizations need an extension of the health system's or public health system's administrative resources, a reliable flow of funds over time, shared recognition in successes, and long-term support from the health system as an anchor institution in the neighborhood. We recognize this must be accomplished by equally recognizing the autonomy, expertise, and mission of the community-based organization. Currently, the social care champions at Eskenazi Health include 1.0 full-time equivalent with a specific focus to develop and sustain community partnerships, although many team members participated in building these relationships.

Information on Best Practices

Best practices exist as consensus recommendations of experts rather than experimental evidence.[1,21] Eskenazi Health benefits from partnerships with researchers from the Indiana University School of Medicine, the Indiana University School of Public Health, and the Regenstrief Institute Inc, among others. A combination of Eskenazi Health resources, local philanthropy, and a mosaic of state and federal funding support Eskenazi Health's role in collaborating with research teams to identify best practices. We monitor the structure and process of care for individual components of the social care infrastructure using existing EHR infrastructure, quality improvement resources, and pilot project funds. Examples include training, deploying, and monitoring the activities of the new workforce, documenting rates of screening and referral for various social determinants of health, and cataloguing the development of new referral networks and resources in the community.

At the level of patients, we also monitor individual patient change in key quality indicators (e.g., HbA1c, blood pressure, preventive health interventions) and couple these outcomes with an accounting of the dose of social care interventions received by individual patients. At the level of communities, we seek to catalog the challenges, opportunities, and successes among potential and established community-based partners, including an accounting for shared extramural funding and related shared resources. This monitoring system is in development. The health system supports $100 000 per year for efforts to monitor the process of the new social care workflows with an additional $50 000 in support from philanthropy.

Summary

Although the cost of this infrastructure will vary across different communities, we anticipate that most health systems would need to invest at least $1 million to $3 million per year to build and maintain this infrastructure for 5 to 10 years. We estimate such a wide range based on the wide range of existing capabilities across health systems regarding social care. Ultimately, we must demonstrate value to third-party payers to engage these funders in support of this work. We do not include this type of program evaluation (demonstrating longer-term improvements in patient outcomes and costs) in our cost estimates. Notably, our cost estimate would also not include the millions of dollars in financial support for the day-to-day operations of social care services potentially supported by the health system to improve food, housing, or transportation insecurity. For example, Eskenazi Health receives approximately $500 000 per year in philanthropic funding to address food insecurity alone, but we do not include this in "infrastructure" costs. In this critical case analysis, we focus on the cost of the infrastructure needed to integrate social care into the workflows and operations of a health care system.

DISCUSSION

This essay describes a critical case analysis of the human capital, operational redesign, and financial investment needed to implement the National Academies' infrastructure recommendations on integrating social care into medical care.[1] This information is particularly relevant to safety net health systems contemplating a greater role in social care. Expansion of care services to integrate social care with medical care requires change in multiple facets of the health care organization. In effecting these changes, we also note that champions of the redesign will encounter cultural debates about the medicalization of social problems and dilemmas about opportunity costs for competing medical care priorities. Notably, a substantial part of this new social care infrastructure must reach outside the health system and integrate the capabilities and limitations of numerous community-based organizations, including the public health system.[22,23] This "bridging" function between multiple organizations requires administrative and communications capabilities not inherently present in the typical health care system.

We explore the challenges and opportunities through the lens of a safety net health system that includes a federally qualified health system with multiple primary care locations in neighborhoods of high need. These are settings where investment in social care offers the best opportunities to improve health. However, state, federal, and industry funding for social care activities in this setting tend to rely on short-term demonstration projects.[23] Short-term funding will not stimulate the costly investments needed for a durable infrastructure. Given the low to negative margins in the overall budgets of safety net health systems, these realities suggest that much of the support for the longer-term investments currently must come from philanthropy. Sadly, the reliance on philanthropy can place the health system in competition with partnering community-based organizations who also seek support through philanthropy and related funds.[22] Although value-based care offers the potential to support the integration of social care in a future state, delivering on the promise of quality, value-based care requires the infrastructure we describe in this report and investments in demonstrating the financial value of these activities to third-party payers.

Although this critical case analysis focused on the cost of infrastructure, there are other practical and cultural barriers to this integration. For example, our community partners seek to raise awareness that social determinants of health and health disparities share common roots in systemic racism, limited educational attainment, and limited economic opportunity. These partners caution against medicalizing these problems and simply growing the resources of an increasingly consolidated health care industry. People want to receive care in their own neighborhood and to rebuild and rely on the strengths of that neighborhood. We hear a strong chorus from community partners that much of this work requires health care providers and their administrative and financial levers to move into these neighborhoods. This colocation in neighborhoods of great need represents a major strength in the current deployment of Eskenazi Health services. Health care systems can best serve as partners and anchor institutions in local neighborhoods by operating in those neighborhoods, hiring people from those neighborhoods, training people from these neighborhoods, and buying goods and services from their neighbors.[20] Economic development is a potent form of health care.

As health systems engage more directly with their local communities, they will of course find that there are many other health care organizations, governmental programs, public health agencies, and faith-based organizations, among others, who also address the social determinants of health. Working toward collaboration across these many organizations equals the complexity we have already described within the ecosystem of a single health care system. High-need patients often put their trust in safety net health systems, the local public health system, and partnering community-based organizations. This is due in part to colocation in high-need neighborhoods, longstanding relationships among these local community-based organizations, and long-term commitment to underserved populations. Third-party payers, as noted by Butler and Nichols, are "learning that effective infrastructure is technology combined with trust, the kind of client trust that community-based organizations and their network curators have and that does not transfer easily to large health plans or new technology vendors."[22(p1245)] In this essay, we focus on building infrastructure within the health care system and building bridges to community-based resources. However, in some neighborhoods, these community-based resources are strained or nonexistent. Thus, investment in the community-based component of the network is also necessary to realize the gains in the investments discussed here.

The NASEM report and other recent consensus reports provide a blueprint for the infrastructure needed to support integrating social care into medical care. While health systems with a robust existing foundation may be able to bootstrap short-term funding to initiate this work, we conclude that long-term investments by third-party payers will be necessary for most health systems to achieve the recommended integration of medical and social care. We also highlight the added complexity and infrastructure needed to grow cross-sectoral partnerships that begin to address the roots of social care issues, including economic development. AJPH

ABOUT THE AUTHORS

Christopher M. Callahan, Amy Carter, Hannah S. Carty, Tedd Grain, Seth L. Grant, Kimberly McElroy-Jones, Deanna Reinoso, and Lisa E. Harris are with Eskenazi Health, Indianapolis, IN. Daniel O. Clark is with the Department of Medicine, Indiana University School of Medicine, Indianapolis.

CORRESPONDENCE

Correspondence should be sent to Christopher M. Callahan, MD, Eskenazi Health, 710 Eskenazi Ave, Indianapolis, IN 46202 (e-mail: ccallaha@iu.edu). Reprints can be ordered at https://ajph.org by clicking the "Reprints" link.

PUBLICATION INFORMATION

Full Citation: Callahan CM, Carter A, Carty HS, et al. Building the infrastructure to integrate social care in a safety net health system. *Am J Public Health*. 2024;114(6):619–625.

Acceptance Date: January 22, 2024.

DOI: https://doi.org/10.2105/AJPH.2024.307602

CONTRIBUTORS

Each of the authors reports sufficient participation in the work to take public responsibility for the content, including substantial contribution to the conceptualization and design, interpretation of data, drafting and revision of content, and final approval of the published article.

ACKNOWLEDGMENTS

We acknowledge the financial and leadership support of Eskenazi Health and the Eskenazi Health Foundation, Indianapolis, IN.

CONFLICTS OF INTEREST

The authors have no conflicts of interest to report.

HUMAN PARTICIPANT PROTECTION

This article is not reporting human participant research.

REFERENCES

1. National Academies of Sciences, Engineering, and Medicine, Committee on Integrating Social Needs Care Into the Delivery of Health Care to Improve the Nation's Health. *Integrating Social Care Into the Delivery of Health Care: Moving Upstream to Improve the Nation's Health.* Washington, DC: National Academies Press; 2019.
2. World Health Organization Commission on Social Determinants of Health. *Closing the Gap in a Generation: Health Equity Through Action on Social Determinants of Health: Commission on Social Determinants of Health Final Report.* Geneva, Switzerland: World Health Organization; 2008.
3. Syme SL. Reducing racial and social-class inequalities in health: the need for a new approach. *Health Aff (Millwood).* 2008;27(2):456–459. https://doi.org/10.1377/hlthaff.27.2.456
4. Weinstein JN, Geller A, Negussie Y, Baciu A, National Academies of Sciences, Engineering, and Medicine, Committee on Community-Based Solutions to Promote Health Equity in the United States, eds. *Communities in Action: Pathways to Health Equity.* Washington, DC: The National Academies Press; 2017. https://doi.org/10.17226/24624
5. Gottlieb LM, Lindau ST, Peek ME. Why add "abolition" to the National Academies of Sciences, Engineering, and Medicine's social care framework? *AMA J Ethics.* 2022;24(3):E170–E180. https://doi.org/10.1001/amajethics.2022.170
6. Farrell TW, Hung WW, Unroe KT, et al. Exploring the intersection of structural racism and ageism in healthcare. *J Am Geriatr Soc.* 2022;70(12):3366–3377. https://doi.org/10.1111/jgs.18105
7. Horwitz LI, Chang C, Arcilla HN, Knickman JR. Quantifying health systems' investment in social determinants of health, by sector, 2017–19. *Health Aff (Millwood).* 2020;39(2):192–198. https://doi.org/10.1377/hlthaff.2019.01246
8. Lindau ST, Makelarski JA, Abramsohn EM, et al. CommunityRx: a real-world controlled clinical trial of a scalable, low-intensity community resource referral intervention. *Am J Public Health.* 2019;109(4):600–606. https://doi.org/10.2105/AJPH.2018.304905
9. Rojas Smith L, Amico P, Hoerger TJ, Jacobs S, Payne J, Renaud J. *Evaluation of the Health Care Innovation Awards: Community Resource Planning, Prevention, and Monitoring: Third Annual Report 2016.* Baltimore, MD: Centers for Medicare & Medicaid Services; 2017.
10. Renaud J, McClellan SR, DePriest K, et al. Addressing health-related social needs via community resources: lessons from accountable health communities. *Health Aff (Millwood).* 2023;42(6):832–840. https://doi.org/10.1377/hlthaff.2022.01507
11. Seawright J, Gerring J. Case selection techniques in case study research: a menu of qualitative and quantitative options. *Polit Res Q.* 2008;61(2):294–308. https://doi.org/10.1177/1065912907313077
12. Crowe S, Cresswell K, Robertson A, Huby G, Avery A, Sheikh A. The case study approach. *BMC Med Res Methodol.* 2011;11(1):100. https://doi.org/10.1186/1471-2288-11-100
13. Institute of Medicine Committee on the Changing Market, Managed Care, and the Future Viability of Safety Net Providers. *America's Health Care Safety Net, Intact But Endangered.* Ein Lewin M, Altman S, eds. Washington, DC: National Academies Press; 2000.
14. Lown Institute. Lown Institute Hospital Index. 2022. Available at: https://www.lownhospitalindex.org. Accessed May 1, 2023.
15. Gottlieb LM, Wing H, Adler NE. A systematic review of interventions on patients' social and economic needs. *Am J Prev Med.* 2017;53(5):719–729. https://doi.org/10.1016/j.amepre.2017.05.011
16. Social Interventions Research and Evaluation Network (SIREN). Available at: https://sirenetwork.ucsf.edu. Accessed July 1, 2023.
17. Little M, Rosa E, Heasley C, Asif A, Dodd W, Richter A. Promoting healthy food access and nutrition in primary care: a systematic scoping review of food prescription programs. *Am J Health Promot.* 2022;36(3):518–536. https://doi.org/10.1177/08901171211056584
18. Pham HH, Schrag D, Hargraves JL, Bach PB. Delivery of preventive services to older adults by primary care physicians. *JAMA.* 2005;294(4):473–481. https://doi.org/10.1001/jama.294.4.473
19. Porter J, Boyd C, Skandari MR, Laiteerapong N. Revisiting the time needed to provide adult primary care. *J Gen Intern Med.* 2023;38(1):147–155. doi: 10.1007/s11606-022-07707-x.
20. Koh HK, Bantham A, Geller AC, et al. Anchor institutions: best practices to address social needs and social determinants of health. *Am J Public Health.* 2020;110(3):309–316. https://doi.org/10.2105/AJPH.2019.305472
21. Commonwealth Fund. Review of evidence for health-related social needs interventions. 2022. Available at: https://www.commonwealthfund.org/sites/default/files/2022-09/ROI_calculator_evidence_review_2022_update_Sept_2022.pdf. Accessed October 1, 2023.
22. Butler SM, Nichols LM. Could health plan co-opetition boost action on social determinants? *Am J Public Health.* 2022;112(9):1245–1248. https://doi.org/10.2105/AJPH.2022.306941
23. Sandhu S, Sharma A, Cholera R, Bettger JP. Integrated health and social care in the United States: a decade of policy progress. *Int J Integr Care.* 2021;21(4):9. https://doi.org/10.5334/ijic.5687

Building a New Generation of Public Health Leaders Forged in a Public Health Crisis

Susan C. Helm-Murtagh, DrPH, MM, and Paul C. Erwin, MD, DrPH

The COVID-19 pandemic presented wide-ranging leadership challenges to public health leaders and public health organizations. In its wake, as the necessity of reconstructing public health and modernizing the Centers for Disease Control and Prevention (CDC) is considered, we reviewed reports from the Commonwealth Fund and the CDC and other leadership-focused literature to identify common themes for a new generation of public health leaders.

We posit that this new generation must have the ability to communicate (build and maintain trust and accountability); forge, facilitate, and promote partnerships; connect public health and health care systems; build information systems that provide accessible, actionable data; engage in systems and strategic thinking and action; center equity and inclusivity and understand structural racism as a fundamental driver and creator of health inequities; and achieve and maintain resilience and self-care.

For each of the 7 abilities, we offer a description, assess what COVID-19 taught us about the necessity of the ability for public health leaders, and offer suggestions for developing (or honing) one's skill set, mindset, and tool set in this regard. (*Am J Public Health*. 2024;114(6):626–632. https://doi.org/10.2105/AJPH.2024.307633)

AJPH June 2024, Vol. 114, No. 6

The COVID-19 pandemic not only placed tremendous strain on governmental public health systems and leaders but invited numerous commentaries and publications calling into question those systems and those who lead them.[1–6] These criticisms challenge all of us in public health to articulate how we can and will build a new generation of leaders in the context of the reconstruction of public health and modernization of the Centers for Disease Control and Prevention (CDC). The purpose of this commissioned essay is to apply our expertise, explained in the recently published book *Leadership in Practice: Essentials for Public Health and Healthcare Leaders*,[7] to this specific challenge.

AN INITIAL FRAMING FOR LEADERSHIP

Two major reports published in 2022 provide an initial framing device for considering how to build a new generation of public health leaders: *Meeting America's Public Health Challenge*[8] (the Commonwealth Fund Commission on a National Public Health System) and the CDC's *Moving Forward Summary Report*.[9]

These reports are complemented by other key contributions to the public health leadership literature that address everything from developing specific leadership skills to identifying critical actions for public health systems to take over the next 5 years and upgrading the Public Health 3.0 framework. These contributions include those of Fick-Cooper et al.,[10] Brownson et al.,[11] Magaña and Biberman,[12] and DeSalvo and Kadakia.[13]

COMMON THEMES FOR A NEW GENERATION OF PUBLIC HEALTH LEADERS

We identified 7 public health leadership capability themes that are common across the Commonwealth Fund's report, the CDC's *Moving Forward Summary Report*, and the just-referenced articles, although no single piece includes them all. We propose that a new generation of public health leaders must have the skill and the ability to accomplish the objectives outlined in Box 1. Drawing from the

BOX 1— Seven Common Themes for a New Generation of Public Health Leaders

1. Communicate: build and maintain trust and accountability
2. Forge, facilitate, and promote partnerships
3. Connect public health and health care systems
4. Build information systems that provide accessible, actionable data
5. Engage in systems and strategic thinking and action
6. Center equity and inclusivity and understand structural racism as a fundamental driver and creator of health inequities
7. Achieve and maintain resilience and self-care

referenced articles and from our own and our contributing authors' work in our textbook on leadership, we offer the suggestions outlined in the sections to follow for building a future public health leadership workforce.

Communicate: Build Trust and Accountability

Leading effectively in the current public health environment requires crisis leadership skills, beginning with the ability to communicate effectively, clearly, and authentically with key stakeholders. From that basis, trust and accountability are formed, strengthened, and sustained.

Drawing from his experiences in biodefense and emergency management, former US Department of Homeland Security official J. Bennet Waters prescribes the following elements of successful crisis communications: anticipation (applying proactive thought and effort to anticipate and plan for events of high probability or high consequence); identification of interested parties and perspectives (understanding one's interested parties and their perspectives and filling information gaps with honest, clear, and frequent communications); clarification (effectively and expeditiously gathering, validating, synthesizing, and communicating timely and reliable information to maximize clarity and minimize the potential for and the impacts of misinformation); simplification (simplifying information without restricting it); repetition (communicating with interested parties early and often using consistent channels); and authenticity (providing honest, authentic information that enables interested parties to form their own fact-based conclusions).[14]

As we have seen all too often in recent history, and as many public health leaders and observers have noted, dissemination of aggressive antiscience rhetoric and mishandling of communication erode the bedrock of trust without which public health cannot succeed. Savoia et al. provided strategies for mitigating miscommunication and misinformation related to COVID-19 from the experiences of 27 leaders in 19 different countries, with an emphasis on "proactive communication strategies, permanent communication task forces integrated into preparedness and response efforts, robust processes to enhance open discussion of controversial topics within government agencies, clarification of how various branches of government coordinate to oversee specific aspects of the overall communication, and development of relationships across public and private entities ahead of a crisis."[15(p86)]

Forge, Facilitate, and Promote Partnerships

Although the mission of public health as defined in *The Future of Public Health*[16] is often quoted ("the fulfillment of society's interest in assuring the conditions in which people can be healthy"), we less often read what follows this, described as the substance of public health: organized community efforts aimed at prevention of disease and promotion of health. Such efforts are impossible without partnerships.

If forging community partnerships is part of the DNA of public health, why is it included in an essay on building the future generation of public health leaders (i.e., don't we know and do this already)? The reason is that forging, facilitating, and promoting partnerships requires systems thinking, and our natural inclination continues to be to "go it alone." DeSalvo and Kadakia were concerned enough with the current degree of partnership development by public health leaders to include strategic partnerships as one of the 5 core dimensions of Public Health 3.0.

The COVID-19 pandemic taught and reminded us that building and maintaining partnerships are critical to public health practice, especially during a crisis. Many local and state health departments needed partners to assist with the overwhelming work of case investigation and contact tracing. Testing for COVID-19 and housing and caring for the homeless required an extensive array of partners, and successful vaccine delivery relied on networks of partnerships.

Many of the case studies in our textbook involve examples of leaders forging partnerships in the context of

COVID-19, for instance transforming community-driven COVID-19 mitigation through a race equity lens as described by Donna Petersen in a chapter on transformational leadership.[17] When Coronavirus Aid, Relief, and Economic Security (CARES) Act money was made available, county leaders worked with a local foundation to identify nontraditional nonprofit organizations that served highly vulnerable communities of color through which aid could be channeled rather than issuing standard requests for applications (which in the past were more frequently responded to by organizations that served less vulnerable populations).

Connect Public Health and Health Care Systems

The efforts over many decades to more strongly connect public health and health care systems are too numerous to count. This is not about filling a gap in meeting the personal health care needs of uninsured, underinsured, and Medicaid clients, as described in *The Future of Public Health* in 1988[16]; rather, it is about connecting individual-level care, which is the focus of health care systems, to the population-focused systems to which individuals belong, which are the domain of public health.

An example of this during COVID-19 is our own experience at the School of Public Health at the University of Alabama at Birmingham, where 2 of our epidemiology faculty members were embedded in the university hospital system, developing and managing hospital-based information systems that were used not only to monitor the daily census but also to track the pandemic and inform decision-making on resource allocation. County and state public health directors did indeed become the "chief health strategists" (as envisioned in Public Health 3.0) in many areas, leading the efforts to match resource availability (intensive care unit beds, ventilators, personnel) with highest needs.

Our own local health officer in Birmingham, Mark Wilson (Jefferson County Health Department), provides an excellent example of acting in this role, as described in a case study on how he managed in the early days of the COVID-19 pandemic.[18] In January 2020, well before the first case of COVID-19 was identified in the state, Wilson activated the incident command structure, allowing the health department to temporarily rearrange its organizational structure and mobilize and coordinate resources (e.g., with respect to subsequent tracking and management of intensive care unit beds and ventilators). This may prove to be one of the most beneficial and, it is hoped, long-lasting impacts of COVID-19: it forced connections between public health and health care systems because, simply, there was no other path to the other side of the pandemic.

The leadership challenge, then, is to build on this momentum to address other areas of mutual concern beyond the pandemic, including addressing social determinants of health, eliminating health inequities, and collectively understanding the roles of public health and health care vis-à-vis climate change and human health.

Build Information Systems Providing Accessible Data

Experiences with COVID-19-related data acquisition at the individual (e.g., case or patient reports), institutional (e.g., hospitals), and systems (e.g., governmental public health) levels have brought to light the many inadequacies of data systems in public health and health care. Much time was lost in having to build and maintain ad hoc data systems because either the necessary pieces did not exist or they were incompatible with other pieces of the system. Some of the integration issues are political, others institutional, and others technical. The electronic data systems used by hospitals are widely varied, and there will likely be little overlap of the health data collected. County and state public health departments' data systems are not connected across states, and there is no integration of national data systems (e.g., the CDC system) with health care data systems.

On top of that, a majority of hospitals and public health entities do not have individuals with the skills necessary to build and maintain efficient data systems or the expertise to conduct sophisticated data analysis for informed decision-making. As described by one of our epidemiologists embedded in the hospital system, too much electronic duct tape and too much bailing wire were used throughout the pandemic (personal communication, Gerald McGwin, December 7, 2021).

The new generation of public health leaders must develop the entrepreneurial skills and be innovative in solving these information system challenges through systems and data integration. Integration of hospital data at the state level is greatly needed not only for COVID-19 but for other health issues, particularly acute events such as stroke, myocardial infarction, and trauma injury. As McGwin further notes (personal communication, December 7, 2021):

> actually getting data systems to talk to each other "under the hood" plus having a user-friendly interface so people with no college training can

> figure out how to interact with the system is the real novelty. The least significant hurdle is the technical one: the true widget is overcoming the fixed mindsets needed to get it in use.

The public health leader who initiates and guides this effort will have to be politically savvy, responsive, familiar with databases and data entry, adept at developing metrics to verify that systems are working, and able to converse with a broad audience.

Engage in Systems and Strategic Thinking

Public health is a complex and diverse intersectoral system. The public health system includes not only public health agencies at all levels but clinical care delivery systems, community-based organizations, private nonprofit associations, educational institutions, private industry, and the media. Each entity has its own role, objectives, desired outcomes, stakeholders, boundaries, processes, and interactions with other players in the system. In addition to being tasked with understanding the attributes and characteristics of each entity, public health leaders must be able to comprehend the relationships between them, the forces that influence their behavior, and how they and the macro-level system are likely to adapt in response to those forces. Only then will we be able to craft intersectoral, collaborative solutions to the thorny problems facing public health now and into the future.

Furthermore, as observed by Holsinger and Scutchfield, because public health leaders are chief health strategists, they must combine the best of both systems and strategic thinking practices if they are to be successful.[19] These practices include developing, adopting, and adapting systems-level strategies to combat the leading causes of illness, injury, and premature death and promote health and well-being; building collaboration between clinical care systems, public health systems, and systems-level allies; and replacing outdated organizational practices with systems-level practices.[19] These are exactly the characteristics displayed by Mark Wilson, as mentioned earlier, in his role as the chief health strategist in Jefferson County, Alabama.[18]

Address Structural Racism and Health Inequity

As Lisa Bowleg wrote in July 2020, COVID-19 revealed—again—the structural inequities that result in disproportionate impacts and risks at certain intersections of racial and ethnic status and class as well as occupation. As long as these inequities persist, she argued, there is no collective "we" and "all"; how can there be when our health experiences and outcomes differ so greatly on the basis of our intersectionality?[20] Public health leaders must concern themselves with the health of all, not only those for whom the system works. It is our individual and collective responsibility to recognize and address the specific needs of marginalized groups. How do we do so?

At an individual level, Corbie et al. found that extended, intensive leadership training that focused on equity, diversity, and inclusion across 4 domains (personal, interpersonal, organizational, and community and systems) resulted in significant gains in competencies related to these issues. Importantly, their research demonstrates that individuals can both acquire and apply the skills needed to achieve organizational and systems change.[21]

At a collective level, in response to the CDC's *Moving Forward Summary Report*, the Robert Wood Johnson Foundation suggested the following considerations to help center equity in the US public health system: taking a holistic approach to equity across the organization and positioning equity efforts for success; earning the trust of communities directly affected by health injustice and supporting community-based health infrastructure; measuring progress and honing strategies according to the experiences of and outcomes among people most affected by structural discrimination; communicating accessibly and strategically with attention to messages, mindsets, and misinformation; and valuing equity when recruiting, training, and evaluating staff and when conceptualizing public health expertise.[22]

An example of a holistic organizational approach to centering both equity and social justice is the King County, Washington, equity and social justice strategic plan.[23] First developed in 2016 and presently being updated, this plan includes goals, objectives, and tactics for 6 key focus areas that span leadership, operations, and services; plans, policies, and budgets; the workforce and workplace; community partnerships; communication and education; and facility and system improvements.

Achieve and Maintain Resilience and Self-Care

Resiliency refers to the ability to adapt to or recover from change; it is sometimes described as emotional toughness.[14] We can think of no better way to express the importance of self-care and resiliency than to quote our colleague, Laura Magaña:

> Leaders need to take proactive, self-protective steps to strengthen and build resilience and reserves. Recharging is an important strategy for resiliency; it is, in fact what allows us to prepare to be resilient. If we recharge our cellphones and computers every day because they lose energy – why don't we recharge ourselves daily, if we also lose energy?[7(p392)]

In her role as executive director of the Association of Schools and Programs of Public Health, Magaña's own need to be resilient took center stage in March 2020. One week before the association's 2020 annual meeting, the COVID-19 pandemic was declared, and the 3-day meeting had to be moved entirely to a virtual platform. "To be able to focus, adapt, and move forward, I had to be resilient, and this helped others become resilient as well."[7(p392)] Magaña's earlier experiences with adversity—an earthquake in Mexico, a hurricane in Puerto Rico—engendered this resiliency: "You don't wait for others, assuming others will act."[7(p392)]

Resiliency has arguably always been a necessity for public health leaders, but COVID-19 demonstrated its cruciality at both the individual and organizational levels. Although there are several factors predictive of individual resiliency, such as self-confidence, self-discipline, and social and family support, it can also be learned and developed through training and practice.[24] Organizational resilience requires leaders to build strong, supportive teams; create a climate of psychological safety; address inequities in the workplace; and understand the limitations of their organization (and their ability to impact those limitations).[24]

CONCLUSION: HOW NEW LEADERSHIP WILL GET THERE

To prepare future public health leaders to respond to the leadership challenges described here, we must expand both our thinking and our actions about how to grow leaders. Although we recognize that many attributes of leaders develop naturally over time, there are clear mechanisms for bolstering, honing, and reemploying those attributes, which may allow for the development of new leadership skills.

First, we need to reinvest in the leadership training efforts of the 1990s and 2000s, as most prominently featured in the national Public Health Leadership Institute. The institute was successful in improving leaders' understanding, leadership skills, and self-awareness; in strengthening their connections to a national network of leaders, forming long-term collegial and supportive partnerships; and in increasing their voluntary leadership activities at the local, state, and national levels.[25] In addition, the institute inspired the establishment of numerous regional, state, and even local organizations that provided leadership skill building and mentorship. These were critically important leadership growth and advancement opportunities, made all the more necessary given the fact that a relatively small percentage of local and state public health leaders have formal educational backgrounds in either public health or leadership.

Second, accredited schools and programs of public health can develop certificate programs in leadership as well as specialized concentrations at both the master's and doctoral levels. This is as important for growing the next generation of public health practice leaders as it is for growing the next generation of public health academic and thought leaders. Such programs will have a greater impact by creating applied leadership academic opportunities involving faculty who have had experience in public health practice. To that end, appointing more "professors of practice" or providing faculty affiliate appointments for local, state, and federal public health leaders will help ensure that students are engaged with practice and thought leaders who can teach from practical experience. Expanded federal funding for schools and programs to offer public health practitioners tuition support—such as through the Health Resources and Services Administration Public Health Scholarship Program[26]—will make it even more possible for aspiring leaders to acquire this type of applied leadership training.

Providing graduate students with the opportunity to foster dialogue on timely public health issues, such as that afforded by the American Public Health Association's Think Tank program, is another way to stimulate engagement and hone critical communication skills for this next generation of leaders.[27] The extent to which academic leadership training for public health can also engage and interdigitate with the academic training of health care professionals (physicians, nurses, occupational and physical therapists, and so forth) can have a significant impact with respect to a shared understanding of language and concepts between public health and health care.

Finally, pairing leadership training for public health practitioners with leadership training for local, state, and federal legislators—such as training available through the National Conference of State Legislators[28]—may open whole new avenues of knowledge and understanding for future public health leaders (and legislators). As abundantly evident during the COVID-19 pandemic, the lack of understanding of the role of other public health actors in response to the pandemic—from the use of emergency powers by state and local public health officials and judicial review of such powers by courts at all levels to the work of state legislatures in crafting new laws—posed limits on the application of leadership knowledge and skills. The same can be said for the "routine" (i.e., nonpandemic) work of public health leaders; support from elected leaders for local and state public action is critical for public health practice.

We conclude by echoing Brownson and colleagues'[11] call for the convening of a National Academy of Medicine committee to chart the path for a new future of public health with special attention to what the next generation of public health leaders will need as they guide governmental health agencies into this future. AJPH

ABOUT THE AUTHORS

Susan C. Helm-Murtagh is with the Department of Health Policy and Management, Gillings School of Global Public Health, University of North Carolina, Chapel Hill. Paul C. Erwin is with the School of Public Health, University of Alabama at Birmingham.

CORRESPONDENCE

Correspondence should be sent to Susan C. Helm-Murtagh, DrPH, MM, Department of Health Policy and Management, Gillings School of Global Public Health, University of North Carolina at Chapel Hill, 1101-H McGavran-Greenberg CB #7411, Chapel Hill, NC 27599-7411 (e-mail: susan.helm-murtagh@unc.edu). Reprints can be ordered at http://www.ajph.org by clicking the "Reprints" link.

PUBLICATION INFORMATION

Full Citation: Helm-Murtagh SC, Erwin PC. Building a new generation of public health leaders forged in a public health crisis. *Am J Public Health*. 2024;114(6):626–632.

Acceptance Date: February 14, 2024.

DOI: https://doi.org/10.2105/AJPH.2024.307633

ORCID iD:
Susan C. Helm-Murtagh https://orcid.org/0000-0002-6193-948X

CONTRIBUTORS

The authors contributed equally to this article.

CONFLICTS OF INTEREST

The authors have no potential or actual conflicts of interest to report.

HUMAN PARTICIPANT PROTECTION

No human participants were involved in this research.

REFERENCES

1. Ward JA, Stone EM, Mui P, Resnick B. Pandemic-related workplace violence and its impact on public health officials, March 2020–January 2021. *Am J Public Health*. 2022;112(5):736–746. https://doi.org/10.2105/AJPH.2021.306649
2. de Beaumont Foundation. Rising stress and burnout in public health. Available at: https://debeaumont.org/wp-content/uploads/dlm_uploads/2022/03/Stress-and-Burnout-Brief_final.pdf. Accessed May 1, 2022.
3. Parmet WE, Erwin PC. The challenges to public health law in the aftermath of COVID-19. *Am J Public Health*. 2023;113(3):267–268. https://doi.org/10.2105/AJPH.2022.307208
4. National Association of County and City Health Officials, Network for Public Health Law. Proposed limits on public health authority: dangerous for public health. Available at: https://www.naccho.org/uploads/downloadable-resources/Proposed-Limits-on-Public-Health-Authority-Dangerous-for-Public-Health-FINAL-5.24.21pm.pdf. Accessed November 2, 2022.
5. Birx D. *Silent Invasion*. New York, NY: Harper; 2022.
6. Lewis M. *The Premonition*. New York, NY: W. W. Norton & Co; 2021.
7. Helm-Murtagh S, Erwin PC, eds. *Leadership in Practice: Essentials for Public Health and Healthcare Leaders*. New York, NY: Springer Publishing Co; 2022.
8. Commonwealth Fund Commission on a National Public Health System. Meeting America's public health challenge. Available at: https://www.commonwealthfund.org/publications/fund-reports/2022/jun/meeting-americas-public-health-challenge. Accessed October 12, 2022.
9. Centers for Disease Control and Prevention. CDC moving forward summary report. Available at: https://stacks.cdc.gov/view/cdc/120813. Accessed October 12, 2022.
10. Fick-Cooper L, Williams A, Moffatt S, Baker EL. Boundary spanning leadership: promising practices for public health. *J Public Health Manag Pract*. 2019;25(3):288–290. https://doi.org/10.1097/PHH.0000000000001004
11. Brownson RC, Burke TA, Colditz GA, Samet JM. Reimagining public health in the aftermath of a pandemic. *Am J Public Health*. 2020;110(11):1605–1610. https://doi.org/10.2105/AJPH.2020.305861
12. Magaña L, Biberman D. Training the next generation of public health professionals. *Am J Public Health*. 2022;112(4):579–581. https://doi.org/10.2105/AJPH.2022.306756
13. DeSalvo KB, Kadakia KT. *Public Health 3.0 After COVID-19—Reboot or Upgrade?* Washington, DC: American Public Health Association; 2021.
14. Waters JB. Crisis leadership. In: Helm-Murtagh S, Erwin PC, eds. *Leadership in Practice: Essentials for Public Health and Healthcare Leaders*. New York, NY: Springer Publishing Co; 2022: 259–274.
15. Savoia E, Piltch-Loeb R, Stanton EH, Koh HK. Learning from COVID-19: government leaders' perspectives to improve emergency risk communication. *Global Health*. 2023;19(1):86. https://doi.org/10.1186/s12992-023-00993-y
16. Institute of Medicine. *The Future of Public Health*. Washington, DC: National Academy Press; 1988.
17. Petersen DJ. Transformational leadership. In: Helm-Murtagh SC, Erwin PC, eds. *Leadership in Practice: Essentials for Public Health and Healthcare Leaders*. New York, NY: Springer Publishing Co; 2022:117–132.
18. Fifolt M, McCormick LC, Wilson ME, Erwin PC. Exploring the preliminary steps of one county health department to manage the COVID-19 pandemic. *J Public Health Manag Pract*. 2022; 28(6):667–673. https://doi.org/10.1097/PHH.0000000000001538
19. Holsinger JW, Scutchfield FD. *Contemporary Public Health: Principles, Practices and Policy*. Lexington, KY: University Press of Kentucky; 2021.
20. Bowleg L. We're not all in this together: on COVID-19, intersectionality, and structural inequality. *Am J Public Health*. 2020;110(7):917. https://doi.org/10.2105/AJPH.2020.305766
21. Corbie G, Brandert K, Noble CC, et al. Advancing health equity through equity-centered leadership development with interprofessional health-care teams. *J Gen Intern Med*. 2022;37(16): 4120–4129. https://doi.org/10.1007/s11606-022-07529-x
22. Robert Wood Johnson Foundation. Centering equity in the public health system. Available at:

https://www.rwjf.org/en/library/research/2022/12/centering-equity-in-the-nations-public-health-system.html. Accessed December 14, 2022.

23. King County. Highlights from King County's 2016-2022 equity and social justice plan. Available at: https://storymaps.arcgis.com/collections/13f70e6fcfd342b287b0b5fc1bb0289c. Accessed January 25, 2024.

24. Harvard T. H. Chan School of Public Health. How to build—and lead—resilient health care teams during COVID-19. Available at: https://www.hsph.harvard.edu/ecpe/how-to-build-lead-resilient-health-care-teams-covid-19. Accessed December 14, 2022.

25. Umble KE, Baker EL, Woltring C. An evaluation of the National Public Health Leadership Institute—1991–2006: part I. Developing individual leaders. *J Public Health Manag Pract.* 2011;17(3):202–213. https://doi.org/10.1097/PHH.0b013e3181f1e3dc

26. Health Resources and Services Administration. Public Health Scholarship Program. Available at: https://www.hrsa.gov/grants/find-funding/HRSA-22-122. Accessed December 13, 2022.

27. American Public Health Association. AJPH Think Tank. https://linktr.ee/ajphthinktank. Accessed February 1, 2024.

28. National Conference of State Legislators. Meetings and training. Available at: https://www.ncsl.org/meetings-training.aspx. Accessed December 15, 2022.

Major Traffic Safety Reform and Road Traffic Injuries Among Low-Income New York Residents, 2009–2021

Kacie L. Dragan, MPH, and Sherry A. Glied, PhD

See also Ehsani et al., p. 546.

Objectives. To evaluate the effects of a comprehensive traffic safety policy—New York City's (NYC's) 2014 Vision Zero—on the health of Medicaid enrollees.

Methods. We conducted difference-in-differences analyses using individual-level New York Medicaid data to measure traffic injuries and expenditures from 2009 to 2021, comparing NYC to surrounding counties without traffic reforms (n = 65 585 568 person-years).

Results. After Vision Zero, injury rates among NYC Medicaid enrollees diverged from those of surrounding counties, with a net impact of 77.5 fewer injuries per 100 000 person-years annually (95% confidence interval = −97.4, −57.6). We observed marked reductions in severe injuries (brain injury, hospitalizations) and savings of $90.8 million in Medicaid expenditures over the first 5 years. Effects were largest among Black residents. Impacts were reversed during the COVID-19 period.

Conclusions. Vision Zero resulted in substantial protection for socioeconomically disadvantaged populations known to face heightened risk of injury, but the policy's effectiveness decreased during the pandemic period.

Public Health Implications. Many cities have recently launched Vision Zero policies and others plan to do so. This research adds to the evidence on how and in what circumstances comprehensive traffic policies protect public health. (*Am J Public Health*. 2024;114(6):633–641. https://doi.org/10.2105/AJPH.2024.307617)

Numerous studies have shown persistent disparities in traffic-related injuries—and in unintentional injuries broadly—by income and race.[1,2] Low-income people are more likely to experience and die from unintentional injuries and face long-term sequelae.[3] They are also more likely to live in areas with roadways conducive to crashes,[4] with low-income Black Americans being especially likely to live in high-crash areas.[5] Despite this, little is known about how metropolitan-area-wide transportation policies affect these populations.

This study uses New York State (NYS) Medicaid data to evaluate the impact of New York City's (NYC's) Vision Zero traffic policy on low-income residents. Vision Zero included a package of over 100 interventions: speed limit reduction from 30 to 25 mph, physical modifications such as protected bike lanes, vehicle mandates such as trailer side-guards, educational campaigns, and traffic law enforcement.[6] Mayor Bill de Blasio implemented the policy in early 2014 through 6 agencies. Modeled on a program established in Sweden in 1997,[7] Vision Zero policies have since been adopted in dozens of US cities, including Boston, Massachusetts; Los Angeles, California; and Seattle, Washington. The majority of road safety professionals advocate Vision Zero strategies.[8]

Traffic-related injuries continue to be a major policy priority, as public concern grows.[9,10] Two meta-analyses concluded that roadway design and traffic calming can reduce traffic-related risks,[11,12] and several studies of standalone interventions, including speed humps,[13] red light cameras,[14] and signal timing,[15] have also found positive

AJPH June 2024, Vol. 114, No. 6

impacts. However, not all Vision Zero packages have proven successful in practice.[16–18] In NYC, reports by city agencies showed initial decreases in fatalities, with a 26% reduction through 2019, yet gains appeared greatest in the earlier years and have stagnated or been uneven for subpopulations such as cyclists since then.[19,20] In the years since the COVID-19 outbreak in particular, reduced law enforcement and riskier driving have raised concerns that NYC may lose any gains from Vision Zero.[21,22] In other US cities, commentators have questioned Vision Zero's effectiveness, citing fundamental cultural and technological differences with the European cities that saw success.[23]

Even if Vision Zero is effective in US cities such as NYC as a whole, it is a nontargeted policy, so benefits may not accrue equitably. Some worry that Vision Zero may increase inequity if high-need, low-income areas are overlooked for interventions, and a 2017 analysis showed that interventions were less likely to be located in NYC's low-income neighborhoods, despite having the highest fatality rates at baseline.[24] Tracking injuries in Medicaid can shed light on how Vision Zero affects low-income New Yorkers and, by extension, whether citywide policies can address injury disparities. Medicaid data provide several other advantages. Most analyses have relied on police reports and Department of Transportation data to quantify changes in crashes,[19] limiting our understanding of unreported injuries, injury severity or sequelae, and costs.[25] Our data capture injuries of varying severity and longer-term consequences, including follow-up care such as physical therapy and medications. Medicaid data enable measurement of medical expenditures, offering an aggregated metric of impact.

Crucially, Medicaid data allow us to construct a compelling comparison group of similar low-income individuals living near NYC—a design that has not been implemented in evaluations to date. Although a recent article comparing NYC streets subjected to the speed limit reduction with those exempt from it found meaningful decreases in crashes, it could not estimate the broader impact of the Vision Zero package, given that even areas exempt from speed reduction still saw redesign, enforcement, and educational interventions.[26] The period over which interventions were rolled out also coincided with other state and national safety initiatives, potentially confounding single-group time series analyses in prior studies. For instance, the public spotlight on traffic fatalities has put pressure on manufacturers to improve safety through backup cameras, collision alert systems, and safer phone integration. Using a comparison group of Medicaid enrollees in nearby areas allowed us to isolate Vision Zero's influence from many confounding explanations.

METHODS

We used NYS Medicaid claims from 2009 to 2021. The sample encompassed individuals who were enrolled in Medicaid at least 1 month between 2009 and 2021 and had a home address in NYC or the 6 surrounding counties generally considered NYC's suburbs (Appendix Exhibit A, available as a supplement to the online version of this article at http://www.ajph.org). Race/ethnicity, biological gender, and county were self-reported by enrollees.

Outcomes

International Classification of Disease (*ICD*) E-codes were used to identify crash-related claims.[27] We included the E81 series under *ICD-9* (Hyattsville, MD: National Center for Health Statistics; 1980), as well as several codes indicating traffic-related incidents of "unspecified" circumstances, and *ICD-10* (Geneva, Switzerland: World Health Organization; 1994) equivalents. The codes encompass injuries involving cars, motorcycles, pedestrians, or bicyclists (online Appendix Exhibit B) and capture inpatient and outpatient visits. To measure traumatic brain injuries (TBI), we modified the Agency for Healthcare Research and Quality's clinical classification category for "intracranial injury" by excluding "late effects" and "history of" head injury and including "head injury unspecified."

Any given traffic injury claim does not necessarily indicate the crash happened that day, as the visit may be a follow-up. To reduce risk of false positives, we implemented a 45-day washout: if we found another traffic-related claim up to 45 days earlier, we counted only the first. Because Medicaid is the payer of last resort, traffic-related claims may be denied if an automobile insurer is responsible for payment. We therefore included denied claims to reduce false negatives.

To estimate financial impact, we calculated Medicaid expenditures associated with the crash and subsequent year of care. We calculated expenditures as the sum of all payments to providers, including fee-for-service payments made by the state and plan-reported payments to providers (for managed care enrollees). It is difficult to determine exactly which health system utilization is related to the injury and which would have occurred even in an injury's absence; therefore, we included expenditures from all categories of care in the 12 months following the injury and leveraged the difference-in-differences methodology (described in the next section) to "wash out" unrelated expenditures (e.g., routine care).

Statistical Analyses

We analyzed the data set at the person-year level: every eligible enrollee had a row for each year, with variables indicating the injury count, injury details, demographics, and months enrolled. We tested for the policy's effectiveness using difference-in-differences (DID) Poisson regression models, with an offset term to account for months enrolled.

We controlled for age, race/ethnicity, and gender to account for time-varying compositional differences between the areas. An interaction term between a location indicator (NYC vs suburbs) and a pre–post policy indicator provided the age-, race/ethnicity-, and gender-adjusted estimate of the policy's impact. We then computed the marginal effects from the interaction coefficient to report absolute risk differences in the outcomes per 100 000 person-years due to Vision Zero, relative to the comparison areas. This DID effect estimate can be interpreted as the policy-induced change in injuries, net of any unrelated trend changes.[28] Standard errors were clustered by zip code to account for varying exposure to different elements of the policy that may lead to nonindependence of errors. Given the pandemic's influence on traffic patterns, enrollment, and utilization, we calculated an effect estimate excluding pandemic years (postpolicy period = 2014–2019), as well as one including pandemic years (postpolicy period = 2014–2021).

The DID design required the comparison group be on a similar trend prior to the intervention but did not require equivalent levels, although we controlled for age, race/ethnicity, and gender in the event that enrollee composition evolved differentially. To build the case that the suburbs are an appropriate counterfactual, we tested the coefficients for each year of the prepolicy period (2009–2013) in a model using dummy variables for each year (rather than a single pre–post indicator) interacted with the region indicator. Prepolicy coefficients close to 0 would demonstrate that the groups were on similar trajectories.

Because we did not have the crash location, we used home address as a proxy. Although some crashes occur outside one's neighborhood, crashes are most likely to occur near home.[2,29] This measurement error would only affect crashes occurring outside of NYC for NYC residents (and vice versa). If a Bronx resident was injured in Manhattan, it would not influence the estimate. To approximate the extent of this bias, we calculated the share of emergency injuries sent to a hospital within the enrollee's county of residence (assuming that emergencies would be taken to a hospital near the crash).

We conducted several robustness checks. First, we focused on 2 NYC boroughs where cars are more common and compared them with the suburban counties closest to them: Queens was compared with Long Island, and the Bronx was compared with counties to the north (Westchester, Putnam, Orange, Rockland). Several other forces were at play around the time of Vision Zero. Most notably, Uber and Lyft rideshares grew in popularity within NYC, increasing the number of cars; rideshares remained illegal in the suburbs until 2017. Second, NYC established a bikeshare program (Citibike) in 2013 that increased the number of cyclists and changed streetscapes. To account for rideshares, we added the number of vehicles registered by county to our model. To account for Citibike, we ran a model excluding enrollees living in the areas where most Citibike stations existed during this period (south of 59th Street in Manhattan and western Brooklyn).

Finally, to address the fact that we could not perfectly identify new, unique injuries for people enrolled in Medicaid for brief stints, we reran the model limited to people enrolled 10 months or longer.

RESULTS

The number of unique enrollees totaled 10 999 419 (65 585 568 person-years). We identified 180 664 unique traffic-related injuries (168 715 individuals) from 2009 to 2021. NYC and its suburbs differed demographically: NYC enrollees were less likely to be White; were more likely to be Asian, Black, or Hispanic; and had a median age 2 years older than non-NYC enrollees (Table 1). Those involved in a crash (in either area) were more likely to be Black and less likely to be female. Subsequent models controlled for race/ethnicity, gender, and age to account for demographic differences that may have varied across the areas over time and been associated with injury risk. People were highly likely to be injured within their region of residence: of people with an emergency injury, 88.3% in NYC and 86.7% in the suburbs were sent to a hospital within their home region. This indicates that most crashes occurred close to home, and any attenuation bias from geographic misclassification was minimal.

Figure 1 shows adjusted injury rates among Medicaid enrollees in NYC

TABLE 1— Medicaid Enrollee Demographics in New York City (NYC) vs Suburbs (Comparison Counties): 2009–2021

	All Enrollees		Enrollees With a Traffic-Related Injury	
	NYC	Suburbs	NYC	Suburbs
Total person-years	51 866 126	13 719 442	140 486	40 178
Unique enrollees, no.	8 585 528	2 413 891	135 244	33 471
Race/ethnicity, %				
Asian	12.8	4.4	6.4	2.7
Black	18.5	12.7	26.1	19.6
Hispanic	18.0	10.6	17.8	8.7
White	13.8	30.6	11.5	28.8
Other/unknown	36.9	41.8	38.1	40.3
Median age, y (IQR)	30.5 (14.1–52.4)	28.3 (12.2–49.2)	30.9 (20.8–46.2)	30.3 (20.5–45.3)
% Female	53.9	54.6	44.4	49.1
Median annual months enrolled (IQR)	12 (10–12)	12 (9–12)	12 (12–12)	12 (12–12)

Note. IQR = interquartile range. Data come from New York State Medicaid claims and encounter data. Race/ethnicity and gender are self-reported on enrollment in Medicaid.

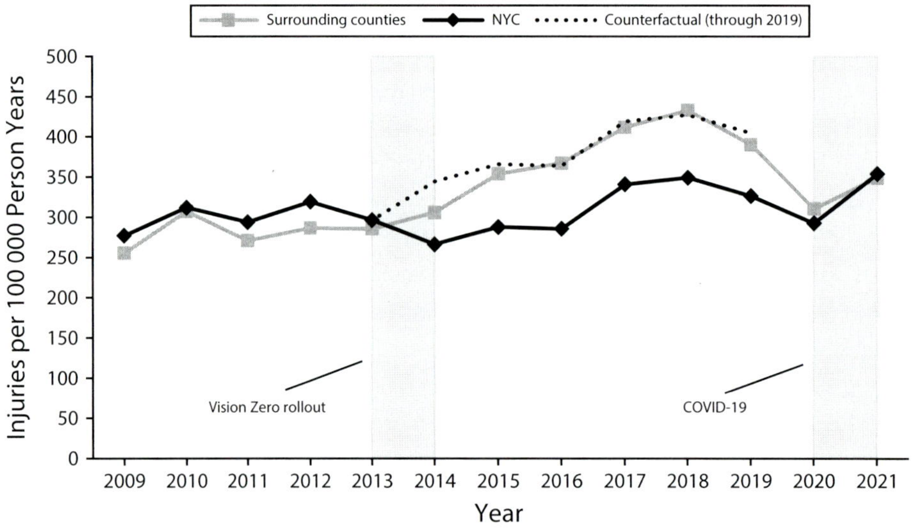

	2009	2010	2011	2012	2013	2014	2015	2016	2017	2018	2019	2020	2021
Surrounding counties	256	307	271	287	286	306	354	367	412	433	390	311	349
NYC	277	312	294	319	296	266	288	286	341	349	326	293	354

FIGURE 1— Adjusted Annual Traffic-Related Injury Rate Among Medicaid Enrollees in New York City (NYC) vs Surrounding Counties: 2009–2021

Note. Rates are adjusted for individual age, race/ethnicity, and gender in a Poisson model with an offset term for enrolled months. The counterfactual line is estimated from the difference-in-differences (DID) regression model described in the Statistical Analyses section: in the absence of Vision Zero, injury rates in NYC would be expected to be 77.5 (95% confidence interval [CI] = 57.6, 97.4) injuries per 100 000 person-years higher than the observed rate. If the pandemic period is included in the DID estimation model, the counterfactual rate would be 62.5 (95% CI = 42.2, 82.8) injuries per 100 000 person-years higher than the observed rate.

versus surrounding counties (unadjusted estimates showing similar results are in online Appendix Exhibit C). Rates in the 2 areas tracked one another very closely prior to Vision Zero, and the DID coefficients for these years (year × region coefficients) are effectively 0 ($P > .05$; online Appendix Exhibit D), suggesting that these counties are an appropriate comparison. Figure 1 shows that the yearly covariate-adjusted rates of traffic-related injuries among NYC Medicaid enrollees were slightly higher than those in nearby counties until 2014 (Vision Zero's rollout), when NYC's rate dropped significantly below the non-NYC rate. This difference persisted until the onset of COVID-19 in 2020, when NYC's rate converged back to the suburbs' rate, reversing the gains from the first 6 years of the policy.

The DID estimate excluding the pandemic years (postpolicy period = 2014–2019) indicates that NYC had 77.5 fewer traffic-related injuries per 100 000 person-years than otherwise would have been expected in the years after Vision Zero's launch (95% confidence interval [CI] = −97.4, −57.6; $P < .001$). This represents a 30% reduction from baseline. Including the pandemic years in the DID estimate (postpolicy period = 2014–2021) gives a total decrease of 62.5 fewer injuries per 100 000 person-years (95% CI = −82.8, −42.2; $P < .001$)—a lower effect estimate, which reflects the reversal of Vision Zero's progress during the pandemic. Online Appendix Exhibit F shows full regression output.

We examined several subtypes of traffic-related injuries to assess whether particularly severe crashes decreased. Figure 2 shows the adjusted trends for traffic-related hospitalization rates, and online Appendix Exhibit E shows the adjusted trends for TBI. Both outcomes show the same pattern as the overall rate: a parallel trend prior to Vision Zero, followed by a relative decrease in NYC after the policy until the COVID-19 outbreak. The impact for both outcomes also reversed during the pandemic. The DID model estimates a reduction of 3.8 hospitalizations per 100 000 person-years (95% CI = −6.3, −1.3; $P < .001$) and a reduction of 4.0 TBIs per 100 000 person-years (95% CI = −6.3, −1.7; $P = .004$) for the model excluding the pandemic (online Appendix Exhibit F). These impacts represent 18% and 34% decreases from baseline, respectively.

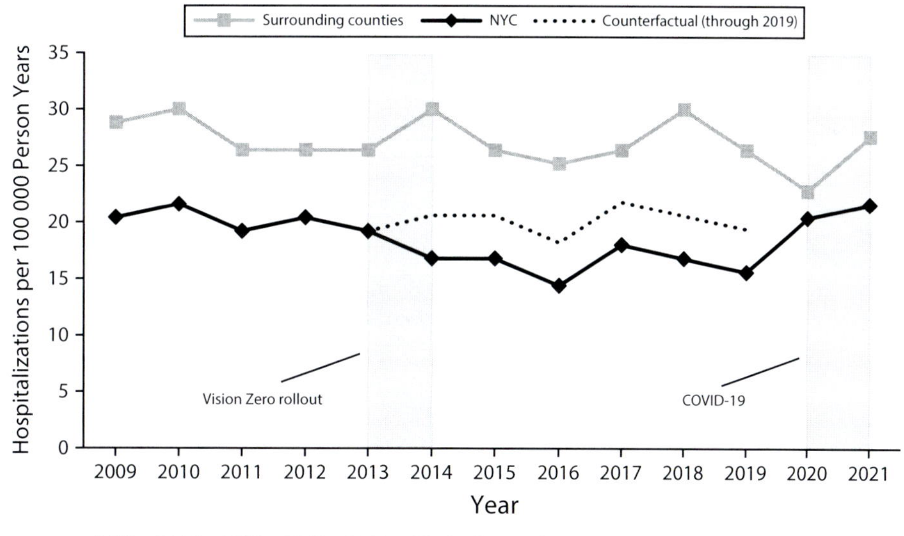

	2009	2010	2011	2012	2013	2014	2015	2016	2017	2018	2019	2020	2021
Surrounding counties	28.8	30.0	26.4	26.4	26.4	30.0	26.4	25.2	26.4	30.0	26.4	22.8	27.6
NYC	20.4	21.6	19.2	20.4	19.2	16.8	16.8	14.4	18.0	16.8	15.6	20.4	21.6

FIGURE 2— Adjusted Annual Traffic-Related Hospitalization Rate Among Medicaid Enrollees in New York City (NYC) vs Surrounding Counties: 2009–2021

Note. Rates are adjusted for individual age, race/ethnicity, and gender in a Poisson model with an offset term for enrolled months. The counterfactual line is estimated from the difference-in-differences (DID) regression model described in the Statistical Analyses section: in the absence of Vision Zero, hospitalization rates in NYC would be expected to be 3.8 (95% confidence interval [CI] = 1.3, 6.3) per 100 000 person-years higher than the observed rate. If the pandemic period is included in the DID estimation model, the counterfactual rate would be 1.8 (95% CI = −0.8, 4.4) injuries per 100 000 person-years higher than the observed rate.

In the model including the pandemic, we estimated a reduction of 1.8 hospitalizations per 100 000 person-years (95% CI = −4.4, 0.8; P = .05) and a reduction of 2.8 TBIs per 100 000 person-years (95% CI = −5.1, 0.5; P = .11).

Prior to Vision Zero, total care in the 12 months following crash injuries in NYC resulted in around $100 million to $125 million in expenditures annually, or around $30 per enrollee ([total spending in the 12 months after crashes for NYC enrollees]/[all NYC Medicaid enrollees]). Our DID model estimates that Vision Zero led to savings of $4.34 per enrollee in annual Medicaid expenditures (95% CI = −8.14, −0.53; P = .026; online Appendix Exhibit F), amounting to total savings of $90.8 million over the first 5 years (2014–2018). That is, had NYC continued to match the trend of the suburbs, total expenditures in the year following a crash would have been $762 million for crashes from 2014 to 2018; instead, actual postcrash expenditures over this window were $671 million.

Given prior evidence of racial/ethnic disparities,[5] we stratified the model by race/ethnicity to obtain group-specific estimates (controlling for age and gender, and clustering errors by zip code). These race/ethnicity-specific estimates show a substantially larger reduction in injuries among Black enrollees (−195.6 person-years [95% CI = −237.0, −154.2]) than all other racial/ethnic groups (−59.4 [95% CI = −82.2, −36.5], −62.5 [95% CI = −87.4, −37.6], and −26.9 [95% CI = −57.6, 3.8] for White, Hispanic, and Asian enrollees, respectively).

To understand the reversal of Vision Zero's gains in 2020, we created a person-month version of the data set. If the gap between the regions was already closing before the pandemic, this would suggest the reversal was unrelated to the pandemic and may have been due to other factors, such as the launch of traffic policies in the suburbs or prepandemic decreases in the policy's effectiveness in NYC. Figure 3 confirms that NYC's reductions in injuries persisted up until February 2020 (15%–20% below the suburbs' rate), at which point NYC's rate immediately converged to the suburbs' rate at the pandemic's onset. NYC never regained its prepandemic achievements (through the latest data in 2021), suggesting that Vision Zero did not operate effectively during the pandemic. This is further confirmed by online Appendix Exhibit G, which uses ticketing data to show that, on average, NYC had 9771 more monthly tickets than the suburbs prior to the pandemic, but had 9715 fewer monthly tickets than the suburbs during the pandemic (DID estimate: −25.4% greater reduction in NYC; 95% CI = −25.7, −25.2).

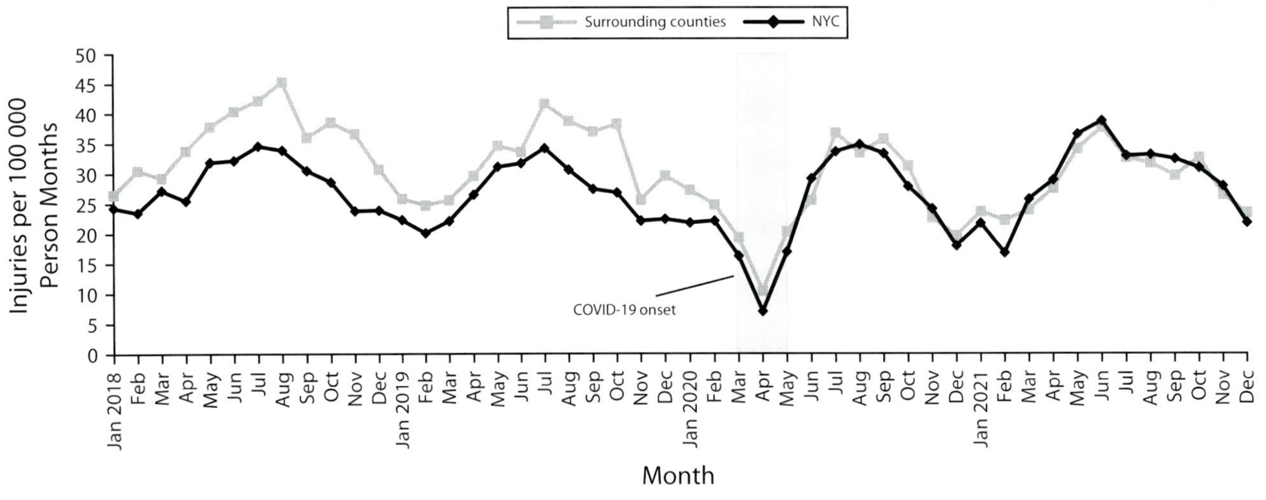

2018	Jan	Feb	Mar	Apr	May	Jun	Jul	Aug	Sep	Oct	Nov	Dec
Surrounding counties	27	31	29	34	38	40	42	45	36	39	37	31
NYC	24	24	27	26	32	32	35	34	31	29	24	24

2019	Jan	Feb	Mar	Apr	May	Jun	Jul	Aug	Sep	Oct	Nov	Dec
Surrounding counties	26	25	26	30	35	34	42	39	37	38	26	30
NYC	22	20	22	27	31	32	34	31	27	27	22	22

2020	Jan	Feb	Mar	Apr	May	Jun	Jul	Aug	Sep	Oct	Nov	Dec
Surrounding counties	27	25	19	10	20	26	37	33	36	31	23	20
NYC	22	22	16	7	17	29	34	35	33	28	24	18

2021	Jan	Feb	Mar	Apr	May	Jun	Jul	Aug	Sep	Oct	Nov	Dec
Surrounding counties	24	22	24	28	34	38	33	32	30	33	26	23
NYC	22	17	26	29	37	39	33	33	32	31	28	22

FIGURE 3— Adjusted Monthly Traffic-Related Injury Rate Among Medicaid Enrollees in New York City (NYC) vs Surrounding Counties: 2018–2021

Note. Rates are adjusted for individual age, race/ethnicity, and gender in a Poisson model.

In robustness checks focusing on Queens versus Long Island and the Bronx versus the northern suburbs, we observed effect sizes nearly identical to the main analysis (online Appendix Exhibit H). To account for rideshares, we added the number of vehicles registered by county to our model. The number of vehicles in NYC increased 12.2% between 2009 and 2017, whereas the number of vehicles in nearby counties increased by just 5.6% (online Appendix Exhibit I). However, after we controlled for vehicle registrations, our DID estimates remained nearly identical, suggesting that growth in vehicles was not confounding the estimate (online Appendix Exhibit H). We also obtained nearly identical estimates when we excluded areas with high Citibike participation, suggesting that Citibike infrastructure was not driving the effect. We also obtained a similar estimate when we limited the sample to those continuously enrolled (≥ 10 months/year; online Appendix Exhibit H).

DISCUSSION

Injuries are an important driver of socioeconomic and racial disparities. We found evidence that in the first 6 years of NYC's citywide traffic safety policy, Vision Zero, the rate of traffic-related injuries among low-income New Yorkers, and low-income Black New Yorkers in particular, fell relative to trends in surrounding counties. Given that low-income and Black Americans are more likely to live and work in places with unsafe roadways and face injuries,[4,5,30] these findings suggest that Vision Zero–style reforms are promising for reducing disparities. One concern with traffic policies is that they affect only the low-hanging fruit (e.g., fender-benders) while having little influence on severe crashes. Our data suggest that this was not the case; residents saw reductions in severe injuries, including TBI or hospitalization. These reductions may have contributed to decreases in Medicaid expenditures. We estimate that Vision Zero saved Medicaid a total of roughly $90.8 million over the first 5 years.

Our most striking finding is that the trend in NYC stayed persistently lower than the trend in nearby counties until the onset of the pandemic, despite growth in crash incidence in non-NYC areas. This finding persists even in the boroughs of NYC that are most like the suburbs, making Vision Zero the most plausible explanation. We explored other potential confounding explanations, including the introduction of rideshare and bikeshare services. Rideshares and bikeshares might increase crash risk, by increasing the number of vehicles and vulnerable riders,[31] whereas other evidence suggests that these innovations might reduce risk because of "safety in numbers" or traffic slowing.[32] However, our results persisted even after we included the number of vehicles registered as a covariate and when we omitted areas with high bikeshare penetration.

Notably, Vision Zero had positive impacts only in the period before COVID-19. In 2020 and 2021, gains from Vision Zero reversed, with NYC's injury rate converging back toward that of surrounding counties. This is not especially surprising, given upheavals to NYC's priorities and density during COVID-19. Two possible reasons include increases in unsafe driving behavior and decreases in traffic enforcement in NYC. Reckless driving during the pandemic—related to increases in driving under the influence or decline of "safety in numbers" in the less-dense pandemic-era city[32]—has been documented.[21] Despite this, the NYC Police Department issued traffic violations at a lower rate than usual in 2020 and 2021, because of a shift in the department's priorities during the pandemic and smaller workforce.[22] Using ticketing data, we found a 25% greater reduction in traffic ticketing during the pandemic in NYC relative to the suburbs, lending credibility to this explanation. This is also consistent with prior research suggesting that speed limit reductions and traffic enforcement may be particularly critical pieces of Vision Zero.[26] Our analyses demonstrate that Vision Zero was highly effective in the prepandemic world for which it was designed; whether it can be effectively adapted to the postpandemic era, and what changes are needed to recapture those gains, remain to be seen.

To our knowledge, the comparison counties did not undergo comprehensive reform, although the NYS Department of Transportation signed the Complete Streets Act in 2011, requiring projects involving state funds explicitly to "consider safe, convenient access" in the design of new roadways.[33] Cities in 4 of the comparison counties made local-level "Complete Streets" pledges for construction involving municipal funds. However, these pledges do not change speed limits or require proactive redesign of roadways, as Vision Zero does. If anything, Complete Streets pledges in some comparison counties would bias our estimate toward the null, only understating Vision Zero's impact.

Limitations

Although our data are comprehensive and the difference-in-differences approach is strong, this study has limitations. First, we did not know the exact location of crashes and relied on patients' addresses. We found that 9 in 10 emergency injuries were sent to a hospital within their region of residence, indicating that bias from geographic misclassification was minimal. Still, future work should leverage better geographic information, both to minimize geographic misclassification and better understand relative contributions of each specific Vision Zero intervention (intersection modification, protected bike lanes, speed reduction) across neighborhoods. Second, we likely missed some injuries because of insurance laws in which automobile insurance is the sole payer. Third, although we adjusted for major demographic characteristics, it is possible that unmeasured time-varying differences in enrollees between NYC and the suburbs could still have biased our estimate. Finally, claims-based coding is subject to undercounting, as traffic injuries are only indicated if providers use "E-codes," which not all providers consistently do.[34]

Public Health Implications

Our analyses provide evidence of a substantial impact of Vision Zero on traffic injuries among a disadvantaged population and imply health care savings. As a cornerstone piece of NYC's recent agenda, Vision Zero generated considerable media attention, and dozens of US cities launched their own Vision Zero plans. NYS's Governor Kathy Hochul recently signed statewide laws making it easier for cities to lower speed limits and increasing fines for hit-and-runs, building on momentum from NYC's Vision Zero.[35] NYC has also recently committed to increasing traffic enforcement to prepandemic levels, suggesting the potential for NYC to realize gains from Vision Zero once more.[22]

Although NYC and other cities continue to face challenges in reaching the goal of zero fatalities,[9,23] our finding that Vision Zero policy bent an otherwise upward trend in injuries supports the idea that comprehensive traffic reform can make a meaningful dent in injury incidence, despite cultural and technological differences with European Vision Zero cities. This evaluation can guide efficient use of resources as the policy evolves and support conversations about why Vision Zero was less effective during the pandemic. Finally, it provides support for traffic reform as a strategy for enhancing health equity by reducing injuries among groups who are particularly vulnerable to the consequences and are at risk for being overlooked in citywide, nontargeted interventions. AJPH

ABOUT THE AUTHORS

Kacie L. Dragan is with the Harvard University Interfaculty Initiative in Health Policy, Cambridge, MA, and the NYU Wagner School of Public Service, New York, NY. Sherry A. Glied is with the NYU Wagner School of Public Service.

CORRESPONDENCE

Correspondence should be sent to Kacie L. Dragan, Harvard University Interfaculty Initiative in Health Policy, 8 Story St, Suite 380, Cambridge, MA 02138 (e-mail: kacie_dragan@g.harvard.edu). Reprints can be ordered at http://www.ajph.org by clicking the "Reprints" link.

PUBLICATION INFORMATION

Full Citation: Dragan KL, Glied SA. Major traffic safety reform and road traffic injuries among low-income New York residents, 2009–2021. *Am J Public Health*. 2024;114(6):633–641.

Acceptance Date: January 26, 2024.

DOI: https://doi.org/10.2105/AJPH.2024.307617

ORCID iD:

Kacie L. Dragan https://orcid.org/0000-0001-9615-137X

CONTRIBUTORS

K. L. Dragan and S. A. Glied made substantial, direct, intellectual contributions to the conceptualization, design, interpretation, and editing of the study and manuscript. K. L. Dragan analyzed the data and drafted the initial manuscript. S. A. Glied secured initial funding for the project.

ACKNOWLEDGMENTS

We gratefully acknowledge the funding for this research from the Robert Wood Johnson Foundation. K. L. Dragan was also supported by the Agency for Healthcare Research and Quality (T32HS000055) and the National Institute of Mental Health of the National Institutes of Health (T32MH019733) for a portion of the period over which this research was conducted.

We thank the NYU Health Evaluation and Analytics Lab and the New York State Department of Health for making the Medicaid claims data available.

Note. The views and opinions expressed in this article are those of the authors and do not necessarily reflect the official policy or position of the New York State Department of Health. Examples of analysis performed within this article are only examples. They should not be utilized in real-world analytic products.

CONFLICTS OF INTEREST

The authors have no conflicts of interest to disclose.

HUMAN PARTICIPANT PROTECTION

This study was approved by the New York University institutional review board.

REFERENCES

1. Cubbin C, Smith GS. Socioeconomic inequalities in injury: critical issues in design and analysis. *Annu Rev Public Health*. 2002;23(1):349–375. https://doi.org/10.1146/annurev.publhealth.23.100901.140548
2. Fung L, Conderino S. Pedestrian fatalities in New York City. New York City Dept of Health and Mental Hygiene. 2017. Available at: https://www1.nyc.gov/assets/doh/downloads/pdf/epi/databrief86.pdf. Accessed December 22, 2022.
3. Kruithof N, de Jongh MAC, de Munter L, Lansink KWW, Polinder S. The effect of socio-economic status on non-fatal outcome after injury: a systematic review. *Injury*. 2017;48(3):578–590. https://doi.org/10.1016/j.injury.2017.01.013
4. Morency P, Gauvin L, Plante C, Fournier M, Morency C. Neighborhood social inequalities in road traffic injuries: the influence of traffic volume and road design. *Am J Public Health*. 2012;102(6):1112–1119. https://doi.org/10.2105/AJPH.2011.300528
5. Raifman MA, Choma EF. Disparities in activity and traffic fatalities by race/ethnicity. *Am J Prev Med*. 2022;63(2):160–167. https://doi.org/10.1016/j.amepre.2022.03.012
6. City of New York. Vision Zero initiatives. 2022. Available at: https://www.nyc.gov/content/visionzero/pages/vision-zero-scorecard. Accessed December 16, 2022.

7. Kim E, Muennig P, Rosen Z. Vision Zero: a toolkit for road safety in the modern era. *Inj Epidemiol.* 2017;4(1):1. https://doi.org/10.1186/s40621-016-0098-z
8. Evenson KR, LaJeunesse S, Heiny S. Awareness of Vision Zero among United States' road safety professionals. *Inj Epidemiol.* 2018;5(1):21. https://doi.org/10.1186/s40621-018-0151-1
9. Staples JA, Yuan Y, Meddings L, Brubacher JR. Are we there yet? The American journey to safer city streets. *Am J Public Health.* 2021;111(9):1586–1588. https://doi.org/10.2105/AJPH.2021.306405
10. Susaneck AP. American road deaths show an alarming racial gap. *New York Times.* April 26, 2023. Available at: https://www.nytimes.com/interactive/2023/04/26/opinion/road-deaths-racial-gap.html. Accessed May 8, 2023.
11. Bunn F, Collier T, Frost C, Ker K, Roberts I, Wentz R. Area-wide traffic calming for preventing traffic related injuries. *Cochrane Database Syst Rev.* 2003;2003(1):CD003110. https://doi.org/10.1002/14651858.CD003110
12. Retting RA, Ferguson SA, McCartt AT. A review of evidence-based traffic engineering measures designed to reduce pedestrian–motor vehicle crashes. *Am J Public Health.* 2003;93(9):1456–1463. https://doi.org/10.2105/AJPH.93.9.1456
13. Tester JM, Rutherford GW, Wald Z, Rutherford MW. A matched case–control study evaluating the effectiveness of speed humps in reducing child pedestrian injuries. *Am J Public Health.* 2004;94(4):646–650. https://doi.org/10.2105/AJPH.94.4.646
14. Mountain LJ, Hirst WM, Maher MJ. Are speed enforcement cameras more effective than other speed management measures? The impact of speed management schemes on 30 mph roads. *Accid Anal Prev.* 2005;37(4):742–754. https://doi.org/10.1016/j.aap.2005.03.017
15. Zegeer CV, Opiela KS, Cynecki MJ. Effect of pedestrian signals and signal timing on pedestrian accidents. *Transp Res Rec.* 1982;(847):62–72.
16. Nelson L. Pedestrian deaths in LA rise sharply but officials remain committed to traffic safety program. *Los Angeles Times.* March 1, 2018. Available at: https://www.latimes.com/local/lanow/la-me-ln-vision-zero-20180228-story.html. Accessed January 16, 2023.
17. The Globe and Mail Editorial Board. 11. Globe editorial: Toronto's road safety program, Vision Zero, is a failure. *The Globe and Mail.* June 13, 2018. Available at: https://www.theglobeandmail.com/opinion/editorials/article-globe-editorial-torontos-road-safety-program-vision-zero-is-a. Accessed January 16, 2023.
18. Leber J. US cities want to totally end traffic deaths—but there have been a few speed bumps. *Fast Company.* August 2017. Available at: https://www.fastcompany.com/3062492/us-cities-want-to-totally-end-traffic-deaths-but-there-have-been-a-few-speed-bumps. Accessed January 16, 2023.
19. Vision Zero Task Force. Vision Zero year 5 report. City of New York. 2019. Available at: https://www1.nyc.gov/assets/visionzero/downloads/pdf/vision-zero-year-5-report.pdf. Accessed May 1, 2023.
20. Fitzsimmons EG. Traffic deaths in New York City drop to 200, a record low. *New York Times.* January 1, 2019. Available at: https://www.nytimes.com/2019/01/01/nyregion/traffic-deaths-decrease-nyc.html. Accessed January 16, 2023.
21. US Government Accountability Office. During COVID-19, road fatalities increased and transit ridership dipped. GAO Blog. January 25, 2022. Available at: https://www.gao.gov/blog/during-covid-19-road-fatalities-increased-and-transit-ridership-dipped. Accessed May 23, 2023.
22. Guse C. NYPD tickets to dangerous drivers down by nearly half from prepandemic year. *New York Daily News.* August 6, 2022. Available at: https://www.nydailynews.com/new-york/ny-nypd-moving-motor-vehicle-violation-tickets-down-vision-zero-20220807-2pkrnnnt7fhmjdvntak3z74q3a-story.html. Accessed May 23, 2023.
23. Zipper D. Why "Vision Zero" hit a wall. *Bloomberg.com.* April 11, 2022. Available at: https://www.bloomberg.com/news/features/2022-04-11/-vision-zero-at-a-crossroads-as-u-s-traffic-death-rise. Accessed January 16, 2023.
24. Armlovich A. Poverty and progress in New York XI: Vision Zero and traffic safety. The Manhattan Institute. 2017. Available at: https://media4.manhattan-institute.org/sites/default/files/IB-AA-0517-v2.pdf. Accessed May 1, 2023.
25. Centers for Disease Control and Prevention. Motor vehicle crash injuries: costly but preventable. 2014. Available at: https://www.cdc.gov/vitalsigns/pdf/2014-10-vitalsigns.pdf. Accessed May 1, 2023.
26. Mammen K, Shim HS, Weber BS. Vision Zero: speed limit reduction and traffic injury prevention in New York City. *East Econ J.* 2020;46(2):282–300. https://doi.org/10.1057/s41302-019-00160-5
27. Ferdinand AO, Menachemi N, Blackburn JL, Sen B, Nelson L, Morrisey M. The impact of texting bans on motor vehicle crash–related hospitalizations. *Am J Public Health.* 2015;105(5):859–865. https://doi.org/10.2105/AJPH.2014.302537
28. Wing C, Simon K, Bello-Gomez RA. Designing difference in difference studies: best practices for public health policy research. *Annu Rev Public Health.* 2018;39(1):453–469. https://doi.org/10.1146/annurev-publhealth-040617-013507
29. Burdett BRD, Starkey NJ, Charlton SG. The close to home effect in road crashes. *Saf Sci.* 2017;98:1–8. https://doi.org/10.1016/j.ssci.2017.04.009
30. Cottrill CD, Thakuriah P. Evaluating pedestrian crashes in areas with high low-income or minority populations. *Accid Anal Prev.* 2010;42(6):1718–1728. https://doi.org/10.1016/j.aap.2010.04.012
31. Barrios J, Hochberg YV, Yi H. The cost of convenience: ridehailing and traffic fatalities. Becker Friedman Institute at University of Chicago. 2020. Available at: https://bfi.uchicago.edu/working-paper/the-cost-of-convenience-ridesharing-and-traffic-fatalities. Accessed January 16, 2023.
32. Getman A, Gordon-Koven L, Hostetter S, Viola R. Safer cycling: bicycle ridership and safety in New York City. New York City Dept of Transportation. 2017. Available at: https://www.nyc.gov/html/dot/downloads/pdf/bike-safety-study-frlandscape format2017.pdf. Accessed May 1, 2023.
33. New York State Dept of Transportation. Complete streets. 2022. Available at: https://www.dot.ny.gov/programs/completestreets. Accessed January 17, 2023.
34. Conderino S, Fung L, Sedlar S, Norton JM. Linkage of traffic crash and hospitalization records with limited identifiers for enhanced public health surveillance. *Accid Anal Prev.* 2017;101:117–123. https://doi.org/10.1016/j.aap.2017.02.011
35. New York State Governor's Office. Governor Hochul signs new laws to enhance street safety, prevent traffic deaths, and crack down on hit-and-run crashes. August 12, 2022. Available at: https://www.governor.ny.gov/news/governor-hochul-signs-new-laws-enhance-street-safety-prevent-traffic-deaths-and-crack-down-hit. Accessed January 17, 2023.

Causes of Death in the Presence of Law Enforcement in Johnson County, Iowa, 2011–2020

Anne M. L. Rempel, MD, MS, Jane E. Persons, MD, PhD, Kate Bengtson, MSW, and Marcus B. Nashelsky, MD

Objectives. To examine sudden and unexpected or trauma-related deaths that occurred in the presence of law enforcement in Johnson County, Iowa, between 2011 and 2020.

Methods. We identified deaths in the presence of law enforcement using definitions from the National Association of Medical Examiners. We obtained data, including demographics, cause and manner of death, toxicology results, and circumstances and location of event leading to death, from comprehensive medical examiner investigative reports.

Results. There were 165 deaths that occurred in the presence of law enforcement: 114 were from a known disease, and 51 were either trauma related or the sudden, unexpected initial presentation of a previously unrecognized disease. Three deaths occurred in the context of physical restraint by law enforcement. Suicide was the leading manner of death among trauma-related deaths; the means of suicide was predictable based on in-custody (hanging) or precustody (firearm) circumstances.

Conclusions. Our findings highlight the potential role of medical examiners and coroners in improving completeness of data on reporting death in the presence of law enforcement to public health agencies.
(*Am J Public Health*. 2024;114(6):642–650. https://doi.org/10.2105/AJPH.2024.307616)

AJPH June 2024, Vol. 114, No. 6

Medicolegal death investigation (MDI) systems, which involve medical examiners, coroners, or justices of the peace, have a unique public service position that bridges the medical, public health, and legal communities. Recognizing the societal value of understanding how people die, US states and territories have created MDI systems by statute to investigate all sudden, unexpected, unexplained, or trauma-related deaths.

A common example of sudden, unexpected death is a death caused by previously undiagnosed heart disease. Common examples of injury-related deaths are blunt trauma from a motor vehicle collision, asphyxia from hanging, illicit drug intoxication, and gunshot wounds. In general, MDI jurisdiction also includes some specific death types (e.g., of those younger than 18 years, from a novel infectious disease, of an unidentified decedent, maternal death, and in-custody death). The outcome of every investigated case is a medical opinion of the cause of death (e.g., a specific disease or injury) and the manner of death (e.g., natural, accident, suicide, homicide, or undetermined).

The work of a death investigation system is centered on public health: learning from the deceased to improve population health and reduce mortality. By investigating sudden, unexpected deaths, trauma deaths, and additional specific types of death as required by law (e.g., in-custody deaths), MDI systems conduct surveillance and generate epidemiological data. Surveillance examples are (1) the recognition and early description of hantavirus pulmonary syndrome in 1993 by the New Mexico Office of the Medical Investigator,[1] and (2) real-time recognition of illicit drug deaths.[2] Examples of epidemiological data generated by death investigation systems are (1) common characteristics of COVID-19 deaths in Cook County, Illinois,[3] and (2) common characteristics of the sleep environment in sudden unexplained infant deaths.[4]

Recognition of MDI as a public health activity is complicated by the incorrect stereotypes of focusing solely on homicide and of conducting an autopsy on every investigated death. Homicides (i.e., injury-related deaths caused by the volitional act of another person) are always medical examiner or coroner cases but represent only a small fraction of overall caseload. Furthermore, medical examiner and coroner death investigations may, but do not always, necessitate an autopsy, which is not the only tool available. The high profile of homicide deaths also encourages a false impression of an MDI office as working for law enforcement. Medical examiner and coroner independence is a core professional principle no matter an agency's administrative placement in government.[5] Death investigation systems do not investigate crimes. Rather, they investigate certain types of death as outlined by state or territorial laws (i.e., sudden, unexpected, unexplained, or traumatic). This independence is particularly important during the evaluation of deaths that occur in the presence of law enforcement. This is an uncommon but not rare case type, and each investigation demands a thoughtful, unhurried approach focused on correct identification of cause and manner of death.

Despite the legal requirement for medical examiners and coroners to investigate in-custody deaths, deaths that occur in the presence of law enforcement are undercounted in the US public health record. This occurs because there is no single comprehensive reporting agency, compulsory reporting mechanism, or uniform definition of law enforcement presence.[6,7] Currently, public health professionals seeking a data resource must rely on a blend of federal- and state-funded programs, including the Death in Custody Reporting Act of 2013 and its derivative, the Federal Law Enforcement Agency Deaths in Custody Reporting Program; the Mortality in Correctional Institutions program; the National Vital Statistics System; and the National Violent Death Reporting System.[8]

Public health professionals seeking to study deaths in the presence of law enforcement are further limited by the lack of a uniform definition in the existing body of literature. Definitions include deaths that occurred in a correctional facility only,[9,10] a specific manner of death or scenario of death,[11–13] and an expanded definition of in custody that includes deaths occurring during law enforcement personnel pursuit or apprehension.[14–16] Relatively few studies have examined county-level data on deaths that occurred in the presence of law enforcement,[10,17–19] and none, to our knowledge, are specific to the state of Iowa.

We performed a descriptive analysis of deaths that occurred in the presence of law enforcement and were investigated by the Johnson County, Iowa Medical Examiner Department (JCME) between 2011 and 2020. We aimed to demonstrate that medical examiners and coroners are key sources of local, case-specific data on deaths that occur in the presence of law enforcement.

METHODS

In a 2017 position paper, the National Association of Medical Examiners (NAME) put forth an encompassing definition of "in custody" that delineates the breadth of precustody and in-custody scenarios of death in the presence of law enforcement.[20] We employed the NAME-defined categories "precustody" and "in custody." We use the term "law enforcement presence" to broadly refer to both precustody and in-custody scenarios.

NAME defined precustody deaths as deaths that occur

> under the perceived or physical control or restraint of a law enforcement officer, a corrections officer (including a private corrections officer), or an authorized employee or agent of a district juvenile secure facility or youth residential facility.[20(p607)]

The NAME position paper emphasized the perception of limiting an individual's "freedom of movement" during the precustody phase and included scenarios in which an individual was in the process of being detained or arrested. Examples were motor vehicle pursuits by law enforcement with the intention of detention or arrest and law enforcement surrounding a house during a hostage or barricade situation. Both examples illustrate that one need not be physically restrained to perceive a limitation of freedom of movement by law enforcement. NAME defined in-custody deaths as deaths that occur while the decedent is "in actual police custody, corrections custody (both pretrial and sentenced), and when the individual is in legal custody but not in the custody of a correctional agency"[(p607)] and defined the start of this phase as the moment of physical arrest.[20]

Medical Examiner Jurisdiction

JCME conducts medicolegal death investigations in Johnson County, Iowa. Although it encompasses only 614 square miles and hosts an estimated population of only 152 854 as of 2020,[21] Johnson County is home to both the University of Iowa Hospitals and Clinics (UIHC), a tertiary care academic medical center that receives patient transfers from much of Iowa and adjacent areas of border states, and the Iowa Medical Classification Center, a correctional facility with medical and psychiatric beds and the only hospice unit for the Iowa Department of Corrections.

JCME has jurisdiction over deaths in Johnson County that are sudden and unexpected or trauma related, as well as over any "death of a person confined in a prison, jail, or correctional institution."[22(p1)] By convention, JCME also investigates all deaths in the presence of law enforcement that occur before the individual is taken into custody. JCME jurisdiction is also determined by the location of death (i.e., in Johnson County) and not by the location of an ultimately fatal incident and, therefore, includes many deaths that occurred at UIHC for which the event leading to death occurred in a location other than Johnson County (e.g., an individual with an arrest-related injury sustained in a location other than Johnson County may be transferred to UIHC for a higher level of medical care).

Data Collection and Analyses

We identified deaths in the presence of law enforcement by reviewing all JCME case files for 2011 to 2020. We extracted data from deaths in the presence of law enforcement from medical examiner investigative narratives, medical records, and autopsy reports, where applicable, to obtain age, sex, cause and manner of death, toxicology results, circumstances and location of events leading to death, location of death pronouncement, and year of death. We obtained the decedent's race through review of death certificates generated using the Iowa Electronic Death Registration System. Funeral homes collect racial identity via interviewing the decedent's next of kin.

We report descriptive statistics as frequencies and percentages. We used χ^2 analysis to compare categorical variables, with statistical significance set at $\alpha = 0.05$. We conducted statistical analysis using SAS version 9.4 (SAS Institute, Cary, NC).

RESULTS

There were 165 deaths that occurred in the presence of law enforcement: 114 (69.1%) were attributable to a previously known disease process, 37 (22.4%) were trauma related, and 14 (8.5%) were the sudden and unexpected initial presentation of an ultimately fatal disease process.

A mean of 16.5 deaths in the presence of law enforcement (median = 15.5; range = 9–28) occurred annually during our 10-year study period. Of the 28 deaths in 2020, 13 (46.4%) were attributed to known COVID-19 disease as either the primary cause of death or a significant infection that contributed to death from another condition (e.g., COVID-19 infection hastening the death of a hospice cancer patient; Figure 1).

Previously Known Disease Process

There were 114 individuals who died in the presence of law enforcement from a known disease process, most of whom were enrolled in hospice (Table 1). These decedents were primarily male (98.2%), White (81.6%), or Black/African American (17.5%) and had a mean age of 62.4 years (median = 65; range = 21–89). These decedents were all in custody at the time of death, manner of death was natural, and none required an autopsy examination because death resulted from a known fatal disease process.

Sudden and Unexpected or Trauma Related

Of the 51 deaths in the presence of law enforcement that were sudden and unexpected or trauma related, decedents were primarily male (86.3%) and White (88.2%). The mean age was 39.4 years (median = 40; range = 13–79; Table 1). All but 1 received an autopsy examination. Relative to those for whom death in the presence of law enforcement was from a known disease process, decedents whose deaths were sudden and unexpected or trauma related were significantly more likely to be younger ($P < .001$) and female ($P = .002$).

The most common manner of death among sudden and unexpected or trauma-related deaths was suicide (n = 22; 43.1%; Table 2). Suicide deaths included 11 (50%) in-custody hangings in which the ligature was a bedsheet (n = 8), telephone cord (n = 2), or jail-issued pants (n = 1). All 9 self-inflicted gunshot wound deaths occurred before the individual was taken into custody and all involved a handgun. The majority of sudden and unexpected disease-related deaths (i.e., natural manner deaths) were attributed to hypertensive or atherosclerotic heart disease or both (n = 8; 57.1%). The majority of accident deaths occurred during motor vehicle collisions while being pursued by law enforcement (n = 5; 55.6%). Among the 5 deaths classified as a homicide, 2 (40.0%) were from a law enforcement shooting (precustody) and 2 (40.0%) were from an incarcerated person altercation (in custody).

More of the 51 sudden and unexpected or trauma-related deaths occurred in custody (n = 30; 58.8%) than during the precustody phase (n = 21; 41.2%; Table 3). The manner of death

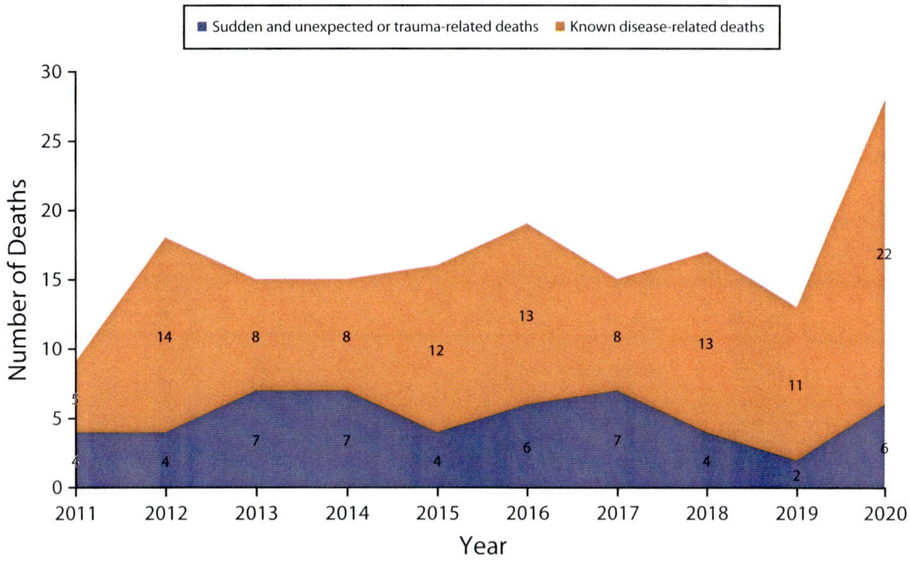

FIGURE 1— Deaths in the Presence of Law Enforcement: Johnson County, IA, 2011–2020

Note. A total of 165 deaths occurred in the presence of law enforcement during this period. Deaths in the presence of law enforcement can be further categorized as sudden and unexpected or trauma-related deaths (n = 51, depicted in blue) and deaths occurring as the result of a known disease (n = 114, depicted in orange).

differed significantly by custody status (P = .002). In-custody deaths were primarily natural manner (n = 14; 46.6%), followed by suicide (n = 12; 40.0%), homicide (n = 2; 6.7%), and accident (n = 2; 6.7%). Precustody deaths were primarily suicide (n = 10; 47.6%), followed by accident (n = 7; 33.3%), homicide (n = 3; 14.3%), and undetermined (n = 1; 4.8%). Among Black/African American individuals, there was a larger percentage of precustody (19.0%) than in-custody (3.3%) deaths. In addition, 3 precustody deaths occurred while law enforcement physically restrained the individual.

TABLE 1— Demographic Characteristics of Deaths in the Presence of Law Enforcement: Johnson County, IA, 2011–2020

	Total (n = 165), No. (%)	Sudden and Unexpected or Trauma-Related Deaths (n = 51), No. (%)	Deaths From Previously Known Disease (n = 114), No. (%)	P[a]
Sex				.002
Male	156 (94.5)	44 (86.3)	112 (98.2)	
Female	9 (5.5)	7 (13.7)	2 (1.8)	
Race				.38
White	138 (83.6)	45 (88.2)	93 (81.6)	
Black/African American	25 (15.2)	5 (9.8)	20 (17.5)	
Asian	2 (1.2)	1 (2.0)	1 (0.9)	
Age, y				< .001
≤ 24	10 (6.0)	8 (15.7)	2 (1.8)	
25–34	15 (9.1)	13 (25.5)	2 (1.8)	
35–44	12 (7.3)	9 (17.7)	3 (2.6)	
45–54	28 (17.0)	15 (29.4)	13 (11.4)	
55–64	39 (23.6)	4 (7.8)	35 (30.7)	
≥ 65	61 (37.0)	2 (3.9)	59 (51.7)	

[a]We used the χ^2 test to compare categorical variables. Statistical significance is set at $\alpha = 0.05$.

TABLE 2— Manner and Cause of Death Among Sudden and Unexpected or Trauma-Related Deaths: Johnson County, IA, 2011–2020

	No. (%)
Suicide	22 (43.1)
Hanging	11 (50.0)
Self-inflicted gunshot wound	9 (40.9)
Exsanguination from intentional manipulation of a medical device	1 (4.5)
Jump from height	1 (4.5)
Natural	14 (27.5)
Cardiovascular disease	8 (57.1)
Infection	3 (21.4)
Pulmonary thromboembolism	2 (14.3)
Neoplasm	1 (7.1)
Accident	9 (17.7)
Motor vehicle collision during pursuit	5 (55.6)
Fall from standing height	2 (22.2)
Complications of ethylene glycol intoxication	1 (11.1)
Complications of methamphetamine intoxication with law enforcement restraint	1 (11.1)
Homicide	5 (9.8)
Inmate altercation	2 (40.0)
Law enforcement shooting	2 (40.0)
Law enforcement restraint	1 (20.0)
Undetermined	1 (2.0)
Complications of methamphetamine intoxication and excited delirium with law enforcement restraint	1 (100.0)

Note. Sample size was n = 51.

For most of the 51 decedents, the event ultimately leading to death (i.e., injury or initial presentation of a previously unknown disease) was not immediately fatal and death was pronounced at UIHC (78.4%). The location of the event ultimately leading to death was most often the Iowa Medical Classification Center (31.4%) or another correctional facility (25.5%), followed by a place of residence (17.6%), in a vehicle either parked or on a roadway (15.7%), outdoors while on foot (5.9%), in a restaurant (2.0%), or at a mental health facility (2.0%).

Postmortem toxicology examination was performed on blood or urine specimens or both collected from 48 decedents in our study and was positive in 21 (44.0%) cases, nearly half of which (47.6%) were positive for multiple substances. Most decedents with positive postmortem toxicology test results died in the precustody phase (76.2%) and were White (76.2%) or Black/African American (23.8%).

All 5 decedents who died of motor vehicle collision injuries during law enforcement pursuit had positive postmortem toxicology test results. Two of the 3 decedents driving a car, truck, or SUV during the event leading to death were not wearing seatbelts. Neither decedent riding a motorcycle during the event leading to death was helmeted.

DISCUSSION

This study provides a descriptive analysis of 165 deaths in the presence of law enforcement that occurred in Johnson County, Iowa, between January 1, 2011 and December 31, 2020. JCME had jurisdiction over every death; it is presumed that JCME captured every death in the presence of law enforcement in Johnson County over the 10-year period. One of our goals was to demonstrate the role of medical examiners and coroners as key sources of data on deaths in the presence of law enforcement. Improving the completeness of data available to public health professionals may improve population

TABLE 3— Sudden and Unexpected or Trauma-Related Deaths by Custody Status: Johnson County, IA, 2011–2020

	Total (n = 51), No. (%)	In Custody[a] (n = 30), No. (%)	Precustody[b] (n = 21), No. (%)	P[c]
Manner				.002
Suicide	22 (43.1)	12 (40)	10 (47.6)	
Natural	14 (27.5)	14 (46.6)	0 (0.0)	
Accident	9 (17.6)	2 (6.7)	7 (33.3)	
Homicide	5 (9.8)	2 (6.7)	3 (14.3)	
Undetermined	1 (2.0)	0 (0.0)	1 (4.8)	
Race				.13
White	45 (88.2)	28 (93.4)	17 (81)	
Black/African American	5 (9.8)	1 (3.3)	4 (19)	
Asian	1 (2.0)	1 (3.3)	0 (0.0)	

[a]We defined in-custody deaths as any death that occurred while (1) in police custody (arrested or detained), (2) in corrections custody, or (3) in legal custody but not in custody of a correctional agency.
[b]We defined precustody deaths as any death that occurred while (1) in the process of being detained, (2) in the process of being arrested, (3) in the process of a law enforcement pursuit, or (4) there was perceived limitation of one's freedom of movement by law enforcement.
[c]We used the χ^2 test to compare categorical variables. Statistical significance was set at $\alpha = 0.05$.

health and—possibly—reduce precustody and in-custody mortality.

Most decedents in our study were male, which is comparable to federal data collected by the Bureau of Justice Statistics and corresponds to the gender distribution of incarcerated individuals in the United States.[14,23] Black/African American individuals constituted 15.2% of all deaths in the presence of law enforcement and 19% of precustody deaths, although only 4.1% of Iowa's population identifies as Black/African American.[21,24] Individuals of color are overrepresented in Iowa's correctional facilities.[25] Approximately one quarter (25.4%) of individuals incarcerated in Iowa are Black/African American.[21,24] Likewise, 23.1% of arrests that occurred in Iowa in 2020 were of individuals who identified as Black/African American.[26]

The overall leading manner of death was natural from previously known disease and, less frequently, the sudden, unexpected presentation of a previously unrecognized disease. These findings parallel those reported by the Bureau of Justice Statistics in a large study of federal in-custody and arrest-related deaths using similar definitions and methodology.[14] It is worth noting that, among all deaths in the United States during 2019 (the most recent pre–COVID-19 year), more than 90% were from natural causes.[27] By contrast, 77.6% of deaths in the presence of law enforcement during our 10-year study were from natural causes. During 2020, the number of deaths in the presence of law enforcement in Johnson County, Iowa, markedly increased because of the COVID-19 pandemic. Throughout the pandemic, incarcerated populations proved to be particularly vulnerable to COVID-19 outbreaks across the United States, primarily because of high transmission rates in prison and jail facilities and the inability to adequately test, monitor, or quarantine individuals in custody.[28]

More than one half of the trauma-related deaths were suicides. Our findings reveal predictable self-injury means among in-custody (hanging) and precustody (gunshot wound) individuals, suggesting the need for future studies regarding improved in-custody suicide risk mitigation in correctional facilities and de-escalation techniques when the subject may have access to a firearm.

Many decedents had positive toxicology test results for at least 1 substance, and most of these were before the individual was taken into custody. All 3 decedents who died while being restrained had positive toxicology test results for methamphetamine. Future studies should consider examining the interplay between intoxicant use and death in the presence of law enforcement.

Limitations

Our study was not without limitations. In data extraction, we used an inefficient manual review of case files (paper and, later, electronic). The proportion of deaths of natural cause was increased by COVID-19–related deaths because of the inclusion of the year

2020. Additionally, Iowa's population has little racial diversity. Given that our findings are specific to JCME, the generalizability of our results beyond southeast Iowa is uncertain.

Public Health Implications

MDI systems are uniquely positioned to recognize, characterize, and report all deaths of those in custody (per the NAME definition) and all deaths occurring in the presence of law enforcement (our terminology). This is because (1) in the United States, medical examiners and coroners generally have jurisdiction over in-custody death cases; and (2) medical examiners and coroners generate a death certificate on every death within their jurisdiction. The death certificate is a well-established tool to collect epidemiological data, and there is a process for implementing updates to identify case characteristics of public health significance (e.g., a new checkbox item to indicate whether a decedent died in the presence of law enforcement).

To an epidemiologist, the death certificate is a survey instrument and data collection device with standard fields and format. Two sections (i.e., "cause of death" and "how injury occurred") are free text and encourage the certifier to use medical terminology (e.g., cause of death) and a simple narrative (e.g., how an injury occurred if not a disease-related death) that together best reflect the certifier's opinion. Other sections are checkboxes or fill-in-the-blank format (e.g., manner of death and date of injury, respectively). Death certificates are state- and territory-centered documents, but all are patterned after a standard US certificate of death.[29]

The standard certificate of death may be updated at regular intervals, with states and territories following suit. The most recent updates of the standard US certificate of death were issued in 2003. Among many changes, the 2003 revision added 3 public health–centered topics: contribution of tobacco use to death, pregnancy status, and general information about transportation scenario deaths.[29] A query centered on deaths in the presence of law enforcement is not among the 2003 revisions.

Medical examiners and coroners should know of every death that occurs in the presence of law enforcement in their jurisdiction and can apply consistent practice to description and reporting. Even though medical examiners and coroners certify deaths in the presence of law enforcement, the in-custody characteristics of such deaths may not be captured on the death certificate for 3 reasons: (1) a specific in-custody query is lacking, (2) the "how injury occurred" section is limited to nonnatural manner deaths, and (3) the free text format of the "how injury occurred" section permits omission of in-custody identifiers (e.g., entering "shot by another person" instead of "shot by on-duty law enforcement officer"). Furthermore, the dynamics and relationship between law enforcement and medical examiners and coroners should be an area of further research, especially when deaths in the presence of law enforcement remain undercounted.

It is likely that an explicit designation of medical examiners and coroners as the source for information about deaths in the presence of law enforcement would yield more accurate data collection for public health purposes. For a parallel success story of medical examiner and coroner reporting, one may look to information gleaned from death certificates during the opioid death epidemic. Medical examiners and coroners have jurisdiction over drug-related deaths and issue a death certificate for each. Position papers have described optimal strategies for investigating, interpreting, and certifying drug-related deaths.[30,31] Following standardized recommendations for how medical examiners and coroners certify the cause of death, there has been a marked national improvement in drug-related death data quality.[32]

There are at least 2 potential mechanisms for medical examiners' and coroners' rapid reporting of deaths in the presence of law enforcement to a public health agency. The first is via death certificates, as described earlier—a strategy that is limited by how the certifier enters data on the death certificate and the absence of a checkbox for deaths in the presence of law enforcement. The second is via a standardized medical examiner or coroner workflow that includes a nondeath certificate mechanism to identify this death type. Optimally, this mechanism would be a component of data collection of every investigated case, whether through a death investigation system's electronic case management system or a state-level electronic death registration system. Either data record system should be programmable for a mandatory query about law enforcement presence. Such a system was added to Iowa's electronic death registration system in 2024 (Dennis Klein, MD, Iowa Chief Medical Examiner, personal oral communication, September 18, 2023). The designation of death as occurring in the presence of law enforcement should be standard practice, as standard as reporting age and sex of every decedent.

Our results underscore the medical examiner and coroner as a key source of data regarding deaths in the presence of law enforcement and highlight the importance of generating a more streamlined process for documenting deaths in the presence of law enforcement. If medical examiners and coroners are tasked with the mandatory reporting of precustody and in-custody deaths in their jurisdictions (via a tailored death certificate or other mechanism), a more complete picture of deaths in the presence of law enforcement in the United States will emerge and provide invaluable public health information. AJPH

ABOUT THE AUTHORS

Anne M. L. Rempel, Jane E. Persons, and Marcus B. Nashelsky are with the Department of Pathology, University of Iowa Carver College of Medicine, University of Iowa Hospitals and Clinics, Iowa City. Anne M. L. Rempel is also with the University of California, San Francisco, Department of Emergency Medicine, Fresno, CA. Kate Bengtson and Marcus B. Nashelsky are also with the Johnson County, Iowa Medical Examiner Department, Iowa City.

CORRESPONDENCE

Correspondence should be sent to Anne M. L. Rempel, 155 N. Fresno St, Fresno, CA 93701-2302 (e-mail: anne.rempel@ucsf.edu). Reprints can be ordered at http://www.ajph.org by clicking the "Reprints" link.

PUBLICATION INFORMATION

Full Citation: Rempel AML, Persons JE, Bengtson K, Nashelsky MB. Causes of death in the presence of law enforcement in Johnson County, Iowa, 2011–2020. *Am J Public Health*. 2024;114(6): 642–650.

Acceptance Date: January 26, 2024.

DOI: https://doi.org/10.2105/AJPH.2024.307616

ORCID iD:

Anne M. L. Rempel https://orcid.org/0009-0001-4229-0873

CONTRIBUTORS

A. M. L. Rempel led the writing of the article. A. M. L. Rempel and M. B. Nashelsky conceptualized and designed the study. J. E. Persons helped with data collection and statistical analysis. K. Bengtson helped with data collection. All authors provided feedback and helped shape the research and article.

ACKNOWLEDGMENTS

We acknowledge and thank the Johnson County, Iowa, Medical Examiner Department, the University of Iowa Hospitals and Clinics, and the Department of Pathology and Pathology Externship Program.

CONFLICTS OF INTEREST

The authors have no potential or actual conflicts of interest to disclose.

HUMAN PARTICIPANT PROTECTION

This work was exempt from institutional review board review (all individuals studied were deceased). Approval for this work was granted by the University of Iowa Hospitals and Clinics Privacy Board.

REFERENCES

1. Centers for Disease Control and Prevention. CDC grand rounds: discovering new diseases via enhanced partnership between public health and pathology experts. *MMWR Morb Mortal Wkly Rep*. 2014;63(6):121–126.
2. Harruff RC, Yarid NA, Barbour WL, Martin YH. Medical examiner response to the drug overdose epidemic in King County Washington: "real-time" surveillance, data science, and applied forensic epidemiology. *J Forensic Sci*. 2023;68(5): 1632–1642. https://doi.org/10.1111/1556-4029.15329
3. Lesnikova I, Obukhau A, Lashmanova N, et al. Report of 5146 cases of coronavirus disease 2019-related mortality from Cook County, Illinois causes of death, demographics, and comorbidities. *Am J Forensic Med Pathol*. 2023;44(4): 285–292. https://doi.org/10.1097/PAF.0000000000000879
4. Shields LB, Hunsaker DM, Muldoon S, Corey TS, Spivack BS. Risk factors associated with sudden unexplained infant death: a prospective study of infant care practices in Kentucky. *Pediatrics*. 2005;116(1):e13–e20. https://doi.org/10.1542/peds.2004-2333
5. Melinek J, Thomas LC, Oliver WR, Schmunk GA, Weedn VW. National Association of Medical Examiners position paper: medical examiner, coroner, and forensic pathologist independence. *Acad Forensic Pathol*. 2013;3(1):93–98. https://doi.org/10.23907/2013.013
6. Feldman JM, Gruskin S, Coull BA, Krieger N. Quantifying underreporting of law-enforcement-related deaths in United States vital statistics and news-media-based data sources: a capture-recapture analysis. *PLoS Med*. 2017;14(10): e1002399. https://doi.org/10.1371/journal.pmed.1002399
7. Corey E. How the federal government lost track of deaths in custody. *The Appeal*. June 24, 2020. Available at: https://theappeal.org/police-prison-deaths-data. Accessed March 11, 2024.
8. US Department of Justice. *Department of Justice Implementation of the Death in Custody Reporting Act of 2013*. Washington, DC; 2022.
9. Brittain J, Axelrod G, Venters H. Deaths in New York City jails, 2001–2009. *Am J Public Health*. 2013;103(4):638–640. https://doi.org/10.2105/AJPH.2012.301042
10. Lozano JG, Molina DK. Deaths in custody: a 25-year review of jail deaths in Bexar County, Texas. *Am J Forensic Med Pathol*. 2015;36(4): 285–289. https://doi.org/10.1097/PAF.0000000000000183
11. Fazel S, Benning R. Natural deaths in male prisoners: a 20-year mortality study. *Eur J Public Health*. 2006;16(4):441–444. https://doi.org/10.1093/eurpub/cki223
12. Gauthier S, Reisch T, Bartsch C. Swiss prison suicides between 2000 and 2010. *Crisis*. 2015;36(2): 110–116. https://doi.org/10.1027/0227-5910/a000302
13. Hemenway D, Azrael D, Conner A, Miller M. Variation in rates of fatal police shootings across US states: the role of firearm availability. *J Urban Health*. 2019;96(1):63–73. https://doi.org/10.1007/s11524-018-0313-z
14. Brooks C, Scott KM, Whyde A. *Federal Deaths in Custody and During Arrest, 2016–2017*. Washington, DC: US Department of Justice, Bureau of Justice Statistics; 2020.
15. Kuchewar SV, Bhosle SH, Shrigiriwar MB, Padole TO. Custody-related deaths in Maharashtra state of India—analysis of autopsies performed at a medical teaching institute during the period 2000–2018. *J Forensic Leg Med*. 2020;70:101915. https://doi.org/10.1016/j.jflm.2020.101915
16. Soyemi SS, Faduyile AF, Sanni AD, Mgbehoma AI, Obafunwa JO. Custodial deaths seen in the Office of the Chief Medical Examiner, Lagos, Nigeria: an 11-year autopsy study. *Med Sci Law*. 2021;61(4): 286–291. https://doi.org/10.1177/00258024211004230
17. Okoye M, Kimmerle EH, Reinhard K. An analysis and report of custodial deaths in Nebraska, USA. *J Clin Forensic Med*. 1999;6(2):77–84. https://doi.org/10.1016/S1353-1131(99)90204-3
18. Lanphear BP. Deaths in custody in Shelby County, Tennessee, January 1970–July 1985. *Am J Forensic Med Pathol*. 1987;8(4):299–301. https://doi.org/10.1097/00000433-198712000-00007
19. Wolf DA. Nontraumatic in-custody homicidal deaths in Harris County, Texas (2015–2019): justification for a separate manner of death category. *Am J Forensic Med Pathol*. 2021;42(4): 363–366. https://doi.org/10.1097/PAF.0000000000000682
20. Mitchell RA Jr, Diaz F, Goldfogel GA, et al. National Association of Medical Examiners position paper: recommendations for the definition, investigation, postmortem examination, and reporting of deaths in custody. *Acad Forensic Pathol*. 2017;7(4):604–618. https://doi.org/10.23907/2017.051
21. US Census Bureau. QuickFacts: Iowa. 2022. Available at: https://www.census.gov/quickfacts/IA. Accessed March 11, 2024.
22. Iowa Code and Iowa Administrative Code. Deaths—reported and investigated. Iowa code §331.802. 2023. Available at: https://www.legis.iowa.gov/docs/code/331.802.pdf. Accessed March 11, 2024.
23. Federal Bureau of Prisons. Inmate gender. March 9, 2024. Available at: https://www.bop.gov/about/statistics/statistics_inmate_gender.jsp. Accessed March 11, 2024.
24. Iowa Correctional System Census. Available at: https://doc.iowa.gov/iowa-correctional-system-census. Accessed March 21, 2024.

25. Iowa Department of Corrections. Racial disparity report, April 2021. Available at: https://publications.iowa.gov/40527. Accessed March 11, 2024.
26. Iowa Department of Public Safety. Iowa Uniform Crime Reporting System. 2020. Available at: https://icrime.dps.state.ia.us/CrimeInIowa/Report/ArrestDrillDown. Accessed March 11, 2024.
27. Xu J, Murphy SL, Kochanek KD, Arias E. Deaths: final data for 2019. *Natl Vital Stat Rep*. 2021;70(8):1–87.
28. Barnert E, Ahalt C, Williams B. Prisons: amplifiers of the COVID-19 pandemic hiding in plain sight. *Am J Public Health*. 2020;110(7):964–966. https://doi.org/10.2105/AJPH.2020.305713
29. Division of Vital Statistics National Center for Health Statistics. *Report of the Panel to Evaluate the U.S. Standard Certificates*. April 2000, Addenda, November 2001. Available at: https://www.cdc.gov/nchs/data/dvs/panelreport_acc.pdf. Accessed March 11, 2024.
30. Davis GG; National Association of Medical Examiners and American College of Medical Toxicology Expert Panel on Evaluating and Reporting Opioid Deaths. Complete republication: National Association of Medical Examiners position paper: recommendations for the investigation, diagnosis, and certification of deaths related to opioid drugs. *J Med Toxicol*. 2014;10(1):100–106. https://doi.org/10.1007/s13181-013-0323-x
31. Davis GG, Cadwallader AB, Fligner CL, et al. Position paper: recommendations for the investigation, diagnosis, and certification of deaths related to opioid and other drugs. *Am J Forensic Med Pathol*. 2020;41(3):152–159. https://doi.org/10.1097/PAF.0000000000000550
32. Warner M, Trinidad JP, Bastian BA, Minino AM, Hedegaard H. Drugs most frequently involved in drug overdose deaths: United States, 2010–2014. *Natl Vital Stat Rep*. 2016;65(10):1–15.

Erratum In: "Impact of a Permitless Concealed Firearm Carry Law in West Virginia, 1999–2015 and 2016–2020"

In: Lundstrom EW, Pence JK, Smith GS. Impact of a permitless concealed firearm carry law in West Virginia, 1999–2015 and 2016–2020. *Am J Public Health*. 2023;113(11):1163–1166.

When originally published, the percentage increase in handgun mortality was reported incorrectly. On p. 1163, the second sentence of the abstract should read: "Firearm mortality was significantly higher (29%) in the years after the enactment of the law; handgun mortality was also higher (45% increase), whereas long gun deaths and firearm sales were unaffected."

A reference was also reported incorrectly. On p. 1166, reference 10 should read: "Planty M, Truman JL. Firearm Violence, 1993–2011. Available at: https://bjs.ojp.gov/content/pub/pdf/fv9311.pdf. Accessed May 25, 2023."

These changes do not affect the article's conclusions. AJPH

https://doi.org/10.2105/AJPH.2023.307382e

Erratum In: "Addressing Health Care Workers' Mental Health: A Systematic Review of Evidence-Based Interventions and Current Resources"

In: Anger WK, Dimoff JK, Alley L. Addressing health care workers' mental health: a systematic review of evidence-based interventions and current resources. *Am J Public Health*. 2023;114(S2):S213–S226.

When originally published, the number of interventions in a randomized controlled trial was incorrectly listed. On p. S215, second column, under Study Design, the first sentence should read: "Most interventions employed a randomized controlled (n = 52; 44%) trial or quasi-experimental design (n = 50; 42%), defined as either (1) a single-group study design (no comparison group) with 2 data collection timepoints or (2) a multigroup study with a single timepoint for data collection (postintervention only)."

The change does not affect the article's conclusions. AJPH

https://doi.org/10.2105/AJPH.2023.307556e

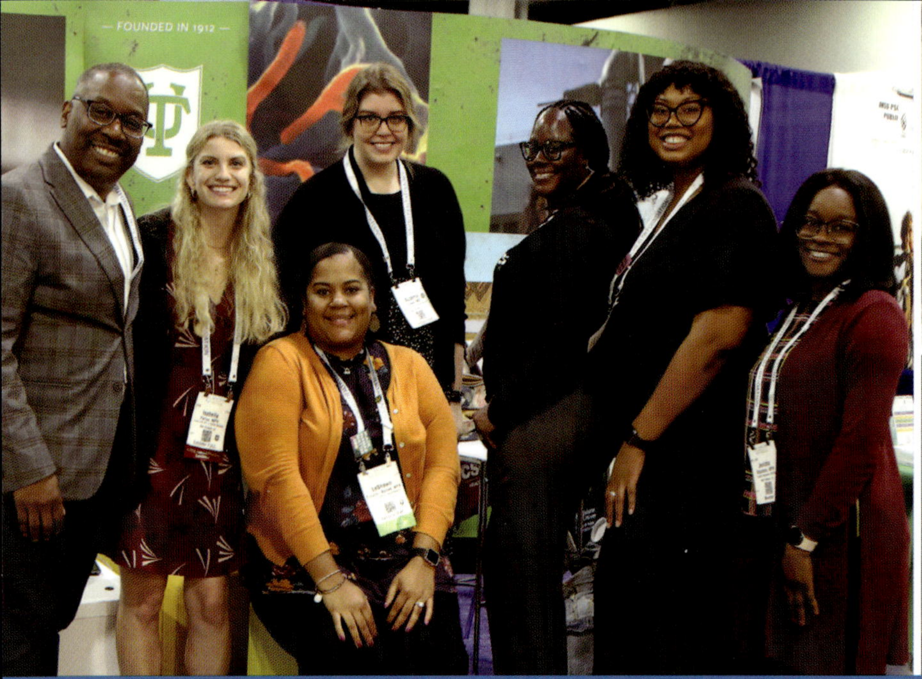
— FOUNDED IN 1912 —
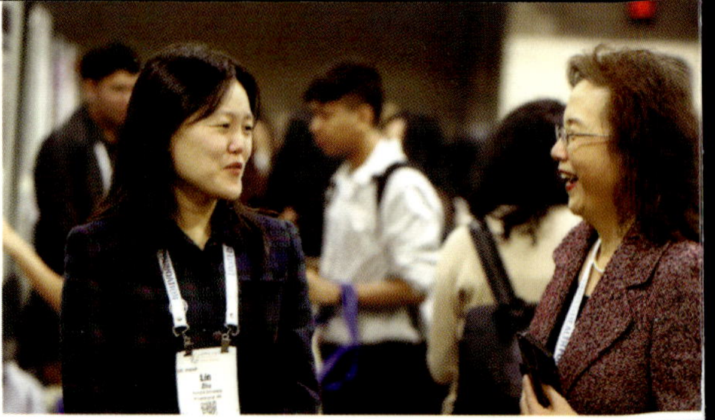
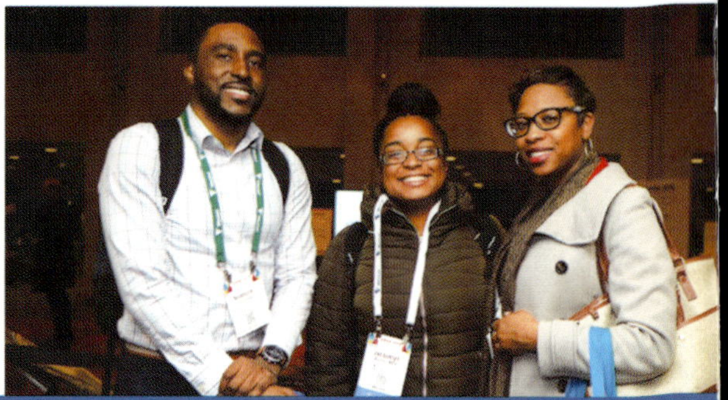